# HISTOLOGY

# PICTURE TESTS

**Alan Stevens** MBBS FRCPath
Senior Lecturer in Histopathology,
University of Nottingham Medical School
Consultant Histopathologist to
Trent Regional Health Authority

**James Steven Lowe** BMedSci BMBS MRCPath
Reader in Pathology,
University of Nottingham Medical School
Consultant Neuropathologist to
Trent Regional Health Authority

Gower Medical Publishing • London • New York

**Distributed in the USA and Canada by:**
Raven Press Ltd
1185 Avenue of the Americas
New York
New York 10036
USA

**Distributed in the rest of the world by:**
Gower Medical Publishing
Middlesex House
34-42 Cleveland Street
London W1P 5FB
UK

| | |
|---|---|
| **Project Manager** | **Claire Hooper** |
| **Design** | **Balvir Koura** |
| | **Tim Friers** |
| **Cover design** | **Balvir Koura** |
| **Production** | **Susan Bishop** |
| **Publisher** | **Fiona Foley** |

Originated in Hong Kong by Mandarin Offset.
Setting on Apple Macintosh.
Output by Text Unit, London.
Text in Helvetica.
Produced by Mandarin Offset.
Printed and bound in Hong Kong.

Cataloguing-in-Publication Data:

Catalogue records for this book are available from the
US Library of Congress and the British Library.


**ISBN: 1-56375-532-7**

# PREFACE

Students enjoy looking at pictures. A carefully selected photograph or a well-drawn diagram is easier to assimilate than written text, and is easier to recall and reproduce under examination conditions. The combination of a clear illustration with a simple written description greatly increases the student's understanding of a topic. For this reason, our textbook *Histology*, published by Gower Medical Publishing, is lavishly illustrated with full-colour photographs and superbly drawn diagrams, many of which are three-dimensional. *Histology Picture Tests* is derived from this parent textbook and is intended as a feedback and revision aid, so that students can assess the extent or limitations of their knowledge of the structure of human tissues and organs. Illustrations taken from *Histology* are used as the focus for questions dealing with important aspects of the subject. Brief answers to these questions are given at the back, together with page references to the parent textbook for more detailed information. In common with *Histology*, we have included questions on the consequences of structural abnormalities in cells, tissues and organs, which are responsible for the production of some common diseases.

We wish to express our thanks to Claire Hooper, Gower's Project Manager, who has bullied us very sweetly into producing *Histology Picture Tests* so quickly after the publication of the parent textbook. We would also like to thank Balvir Koura for her excellent design, and Tim Friers for his supreme efforts in getting the book produced on time. Finally, we would like to thank Fiona Foley, UK Managing Director of Gower Medical Publishing, for encouraging us to produce this book, which we regard as a vital support to the main textbook. We are also very grateful to Gower for the provision of numerous 'working lunches'!

**Alan Stevens**
**Jim Lowe**

# CONTENTS

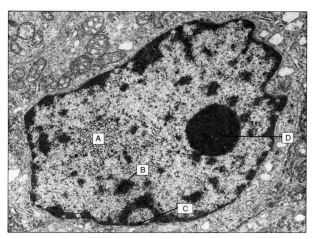

**Q1.** In this electron micrograph of a cell nucleus, what are the terms given to the pale **A** and dark **B** areas of chromatin?

**Q2.** What is present at the nuclear boundary **C**?

**Q3.** What is structure **D**?

**Q4.** What is the function of structure **D**?

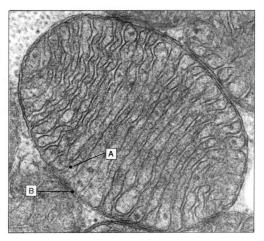

**Q5.** Identify the structure seen in this high power electron micrograph.

**Q6.** What functions are carried out on the outer membrane **B**?

**Q7.** What name is given to structures formed by the folded inner membrane **A**?

**Q8.** How are mitochondrial proteins made?

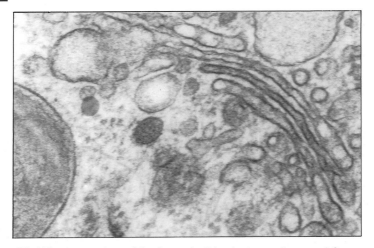

·**Q9.** What area of a cell is shown in this electron micrograph?

**Q10.** What are its main functions?

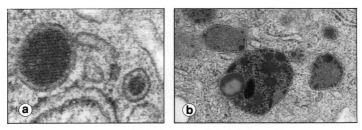

**Q11.** Identify the organelles seen in high power electron micrographs (a) and (b).

**Q12.** What is their function?

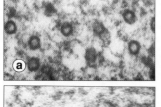

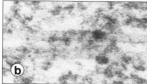

**Q13.** Identify the cytoskeletal structures seen in (a) cross section and (b) longitudinal section in these electron micrographs.

**Q14.** What are the main proteins forming these structures?

**Q15.** What are the other two main cytoskeletal filaments?

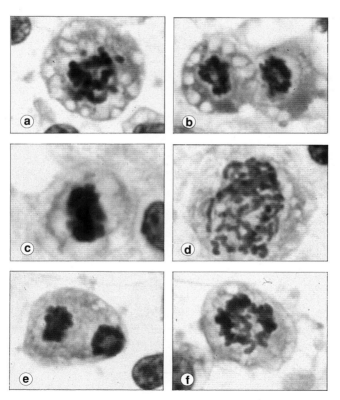

**Q16.** Identify the stages **A-F** in cell division and give the correct sequence.

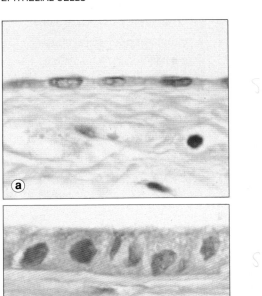

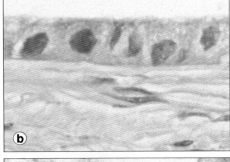

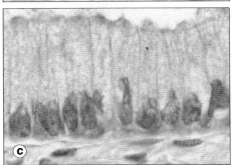

Simple
Squamous

Simple
Cuboidal

Simple
columnar

**Q17.** Identify the epithelial types shown in micrographs (a), (b) and (c).

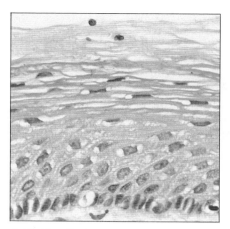

**Q18.** Identify the type of epithelium shown in this micrograph.

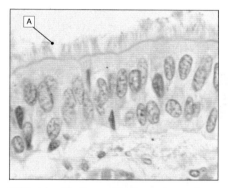

**Q19.** Identify the epithelium shown here.

**Q20.** What structures form the layer **A**?

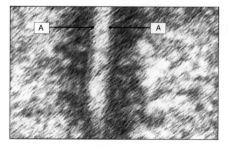

**Q21.** This is an electron micrograph of an occluding junction between cells. What is the term given to describe the arrangements of membrane proteins in the electron dense areas **A** which hold the cells together?

**Q22.** What are the two main functions of such junctions?

**Q23.** What is an alternative name for occluding junctions?

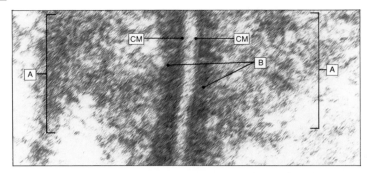

**Q24.** This is an electron micrograph of an adherent junction between adjacent cells. What filaments **A** are linked in this type of junction?

**Q25.** What proteins are present in the attachment plaque **B** adjacent to the cell membrane **CM**?

**Q26.** What other type of junction has the same filament type as is present in adherent junctions?

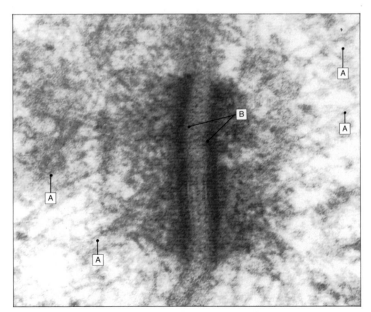

**Q27.** This is an electron micrograph of a desmosomal junction between cells. What filaments **A** are attached to the desmosome?

**Q28.** What is the name given to the electron dense areas **B**?

**Q29.** What is the function of this type of junction?

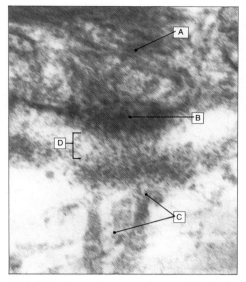

**Q30.** This is an electron micrograph of a hemidesmosome. What is the function of this type of cell junction?

**Q31.** What filaments **A** in cells are linked to the junction via the dense plaque **B** and anchoring filaments **D**?

**Q32.** What is the composition of the banded anchoring fibrils **C**?

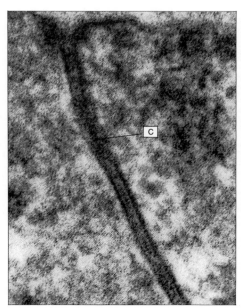

**Q33.** This is an electron micrograph of a communicating junction between adjacent cells. What structures, labelled **C**, does this type of junction have traversing the cell membrane?

**Q34.** Which tissues contain numerous communicating junctions?

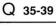

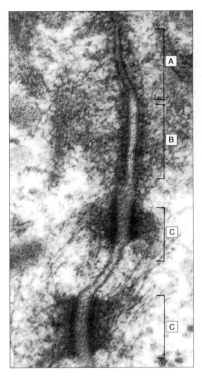

**Q35.** This is an electron micrograph of adjacent cells that are united by a series of junctions. What is the term used to describe such an area?

**Q36.** Identify the different junctions **A**-**C**.

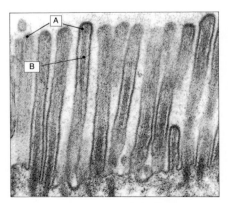

**Q37.** Identify the cell surface specialization **A** shown in this electron micrograph?

**Q38.** What is the composition of the filaments **B**?

**Q39.** What is located in the cell membrane of these structures?

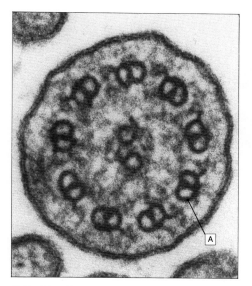

**Q40.** Identify the structure shown in this electron micrograph.

**Q41.** What is the main protein that forms structure **A**?

**Q42.** What term is applied to this cytoskeletal arrangement?

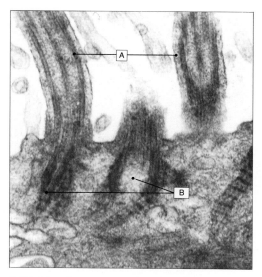

**Q43.** Identify the structures **A** arising from the cell surface?

**Q44.** What is structure **B**?

**Q45.** From what cellular organelle is structure **B** derived?

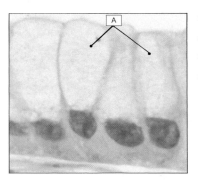

**Q46.** This electron micrograph is of an abnormally formed cilium from a person with a genetic defect resulting in defective cilial function. What is abnormal about structures **A**?

**Q47.** What defective functions would be expected in a person with abnormal cilia?

**Q48.** Identify the product **A** secreted by these cells.

**Q49.** What are these cells called?

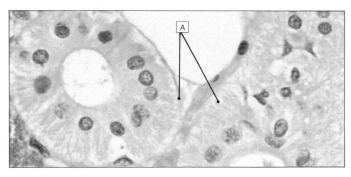

**Q50.** For what function are the cells **A** in these ducts specialized?

**Q51.** What features point to this specialization?

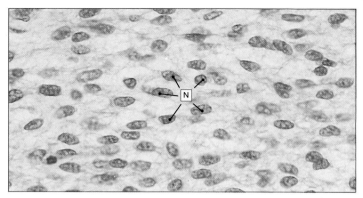

**Q52.** What is the name given to this embryonic tissue, characterized by spindle-shaped cells with large nuclei **N**, from which support cells are derived?

**Q53.** What are the two main components of the extracellular matrix of support tissues?

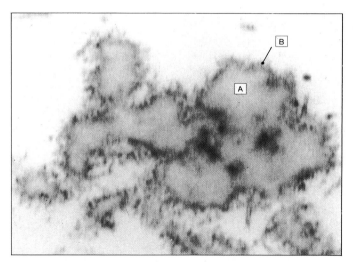

**Q54.** In this electron micrograph of an elastic fibre, what are areas **A** and **B** composed of?

**Q55.** What type of cells produce elastin?

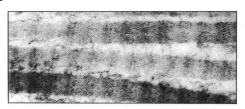

**Q56.** What is responsible for the ultrastructural banding of collagen fibrils, as shown in this electron micrograph?

**Q57.** What are reticular fibres?

**Q58.** Where is type IV collagen found?

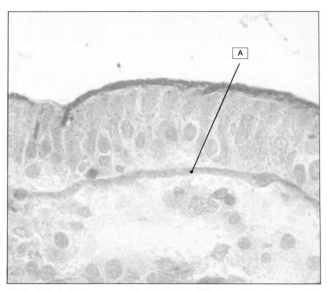

**Q59.** What is the structure **A** at the interface between epithelium and support tissue?

**Q60.** What are its main constituents?

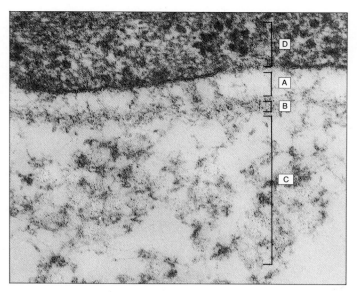

**Q61.** Identify the layers **A-C** of the basement membrane, attached to an epithelial cell **D,** in this electron micrograph.

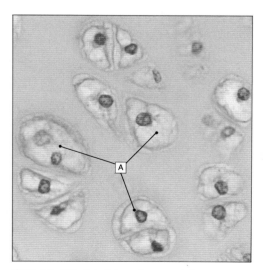

**Q62.** Identify this type of support tissue.

**Q63.** What is the composition of the extracellular matrix?

**Q64.** What is the name of the cells labelled **A**?

**Q65.** Name the three specialized types of this tissue.

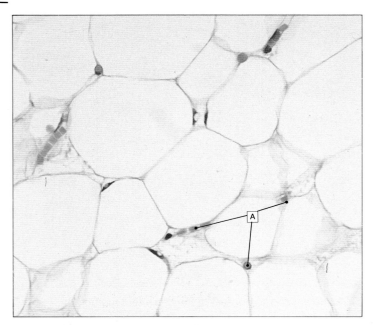

**Q66.** Identify this type of support tissue.

**Q67.** What are the structures labelled **A**?

**Q68.** What are the two main functions of this tissue?

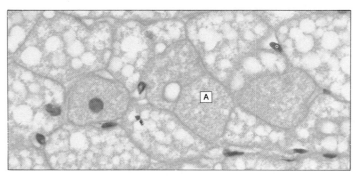

**Q69.** Identify this tissue.

**Q70.** What is responsible for the granular pink staining of the cells labelled **A**?

**Q71.** What is the function of this tissue?

**Q72.** What is its alternative name?

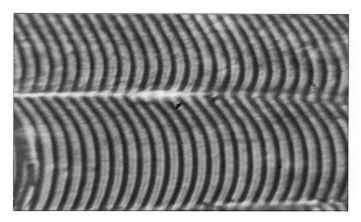

**Q73.** Identify this tissue.

**Q74.** How is this tissue formed in embryogenesis?

**Q75.** What special terms are used to describe the cell membrane, cytoplasm and endoplasmic reticulum of this cell type?

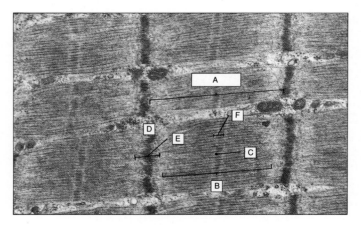

**Q76.** Identify structures **A-F** in this electron micrograph of skeletal muscle.

**Q77.** What filamentous protein forms the structure **B**?

**Q78.** What filamentous protein forms the structure **E**?

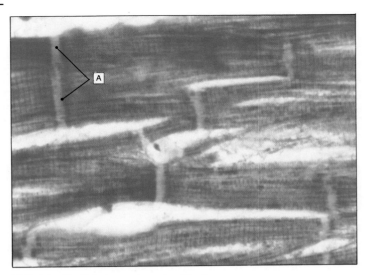

**Q79.** Identify this type of contractile tissue.

**Q80.** Identify structure **A**.

**Q81.** What is the structure and function of **A**?

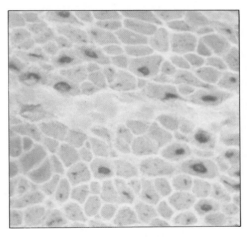

**Q82.** Identify the type of contractile tissue shown here in transverse section.

**Q83.** What surrounds each cell?

**Q84.** How are adjacent cells connected to facilitate membrane excitation?

**Q85.** What intermediate filament is special to this cell type?

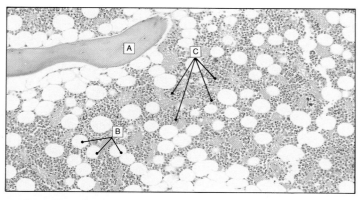

**Q86.** Identify this tissue.

**Q87.** Identify the components labelled **A**-**C**.

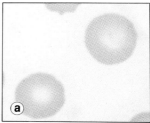

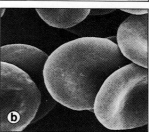

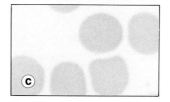

**Q88.** Identify the cells shown in (a) and (b).

**Q89.** What is wrong with their abnormal equivalent shown in (c)?

**Q90.** What is the name of this disorder, and what is its cause?

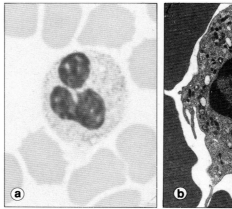
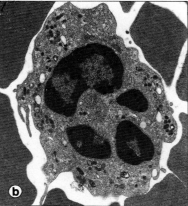

(a)     (b)

**Q91.** Identify the type of circulating white blood cell shown in (a) and (b).

**Q92.** How many nuclei does it contain?

**Q93.** What is the function of this cell type?

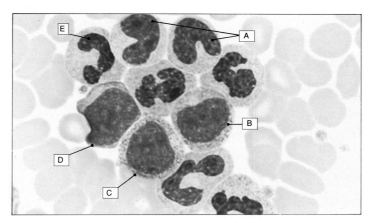

**Q94.** This cluster of cells contain the precursors of mature neutrophil granulocytes - the myeloblast, promyelocyte, myelocyte, metamyelocyte and stab form. Match them with the cells labelled **A-E**.

**Q95.** Where does neutrophil formation take place?

**Q96.** In cancerous proliferation of this cell line, abnormal neutrophil precursors appear in the circulating blood. What name is given to these diseases?

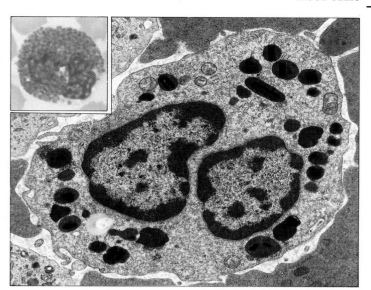

**Q97.** Identify this white blood cell.

**Q98.** How many nuclei does it have?

**Q99.** What is its major cytoplasmic organelle?

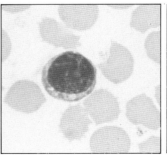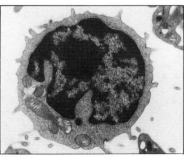

**Q100.** Identify this type of white blood cell.

**Q101.** What are its main functions?

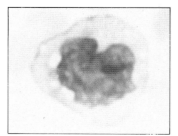

**Q102.** Identify this type of white blood cell.

**Q103.** What does it become when it enters the tissues?

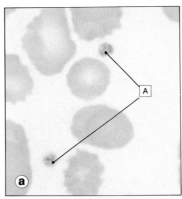

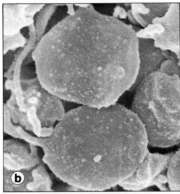

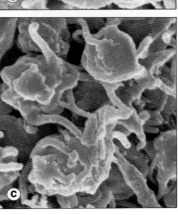

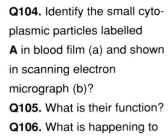

**Q104.** Identify the small cytoplasmic particles labelled **A** in blood film (a) and shown in scanning electron micrograph (b)?

**Q105.** What is their function?

**Q106.** What is happening to them in (c)?

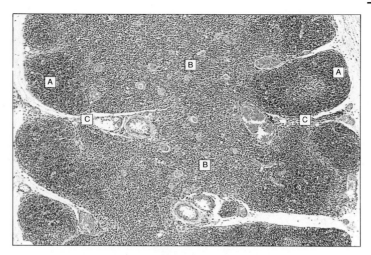

**Q107.** Identify the regions on the thymus labelled **A**-**C**.

**Q108.** What are the four main cell types in the thymus?

**Q109.** What are the functions of the thymic epitheliocytes?

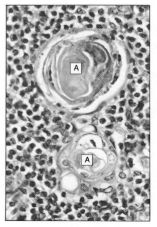

**Q110.** Identify the structures labelled **A** in the thymus gland.

**Q111.** What cells are they derived from?

**Q112.** In what region of the thymus are they found?

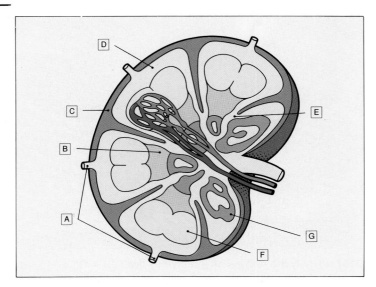

**Q113.** Identify the structures labelled **A**-**G** in this diagram of a lymph node.

**Q114.** What is the predominant type of lymphocyte in **F**?

**Q115.** What is the predominant type of lymphocyte in **B**?

**Q116.** By what route do most lymphocytes enter the node?

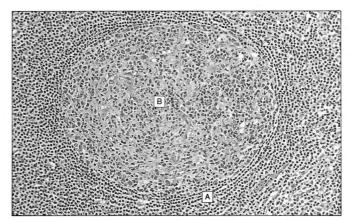

**Q117.** Identify zones **A** and **B** in this structure from a lymph node.

**Q118.** What are the main cell types in this nodal region?

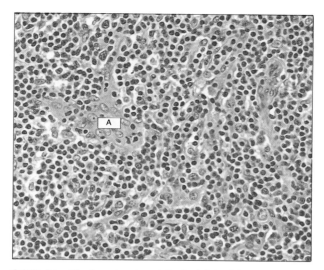

**Q119.** Identify the structure labelled **A** in this area of lymph node paracortex?

**Q120.** What is the function of structure **A**?

**Q121.** What are the main cell types in the paracortex?

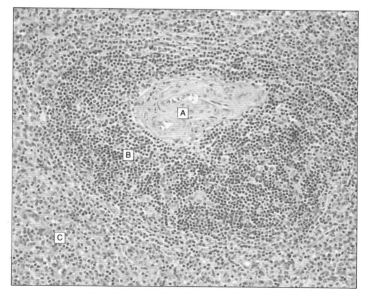

**Q122.** Identify the structure **A** and areas **B** and **C** in this micrograph of a portion of spleen.

**Q123.** What are the two main functions of the spleen?

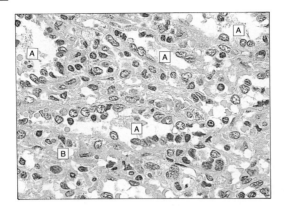

**Q124.** Identify structures **A** and **B** in this micrograph of the red pulp of the spleen.

**Q125.** What cells line structure **A**?

**Q126.** What is structure **B** composed of?

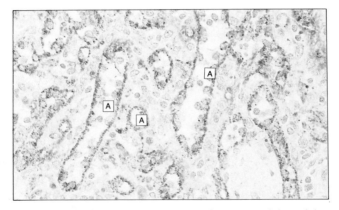

**Q127.** This micrograph shows brown immunostaining of the phagocytic cells **A** associated with the red pulp sinuses of the spleen. What is the structure of the walls of these sinuses?

**Q128.** What is the function of these phagocytic cells?

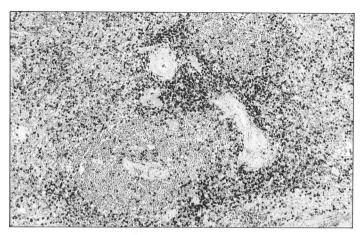

**Q129.** This micrograph shows splenic white pulp immunostained to detect a certain type of lymphoid cell. Which type is demonstrated?

**Q130.** What is the function of the perilymphoid zone, immediately surrounding the white pulp, in the spleen?

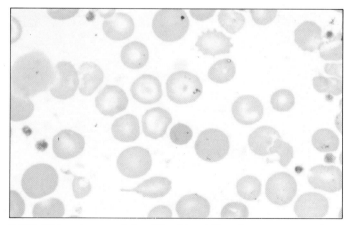

**Q131.** This micrograph is of the blood film of a person who has had a splenectomy. What abnormalities are seen?

**Q132.** What effect does splenectomy have on immune function?

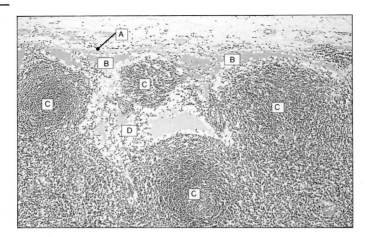

**Q133.** Identify the structures and areas labelled **A**-**D** in this portion of lymph node.

**Q134.** What is the main site of entry of lymphocytes into the node?

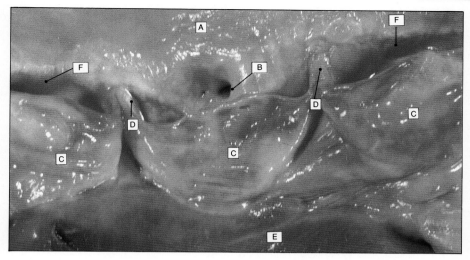

**Q135.** Identify the structures **A-F** in this photograph of the aortic valve.

**Q136.** What originates at **B**?

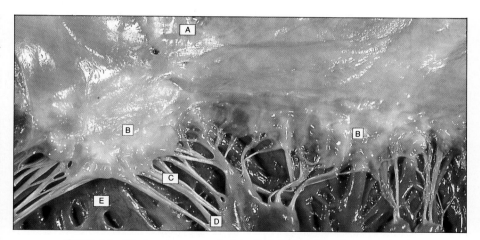

**Q137.** Identify the components labelled **A-E** in this photograph of the left atrioventricular (mitral) valves.

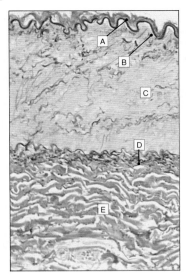

**Q138.** This photomicrograph shows the wall of a muscular artery, stained by a method which stains elastic fibres black, smooth muscle yellow and collagen red. Identify the structures **A-E**.

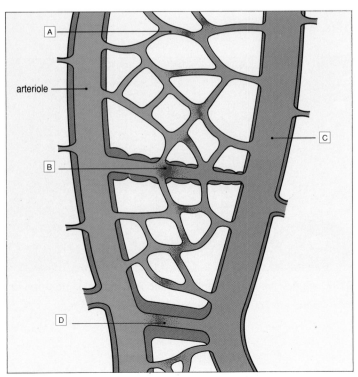

**Q139.** In this diagram of the blood microcirculation, the arteriole is labelled. Identify the components labelled **A-D**.

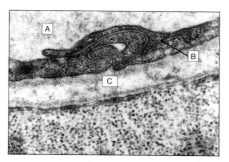

**Q140.** This electron micrograph shows part of the wall of a capillary. Identify the structures labelled **A**-**C**.

**Q141.** What are the characteristic cytoplasmic organelles of **B**?

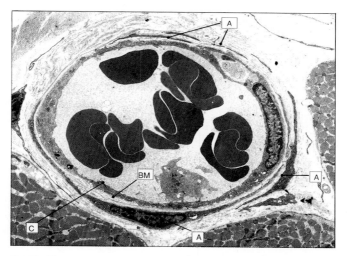

**Q142.** This electron micrograph of a small post-capillary venule shows the endothelial cell cytoplasm **C** and basement membrane **BM**. Identify the narrow cells labelled **A** around the periphery of the vessel?

**Q143.** What is their function?

**Q144.** In larger venules, what are these cells replaced by?

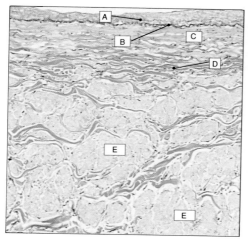

**Q145.** This micrograph shows the wall of the inferior vena cava, the largest vein in the body, stained by a method which stains elastic fibres black, smooth muscle yellow and collagen red. Identify the structures **A-E**.

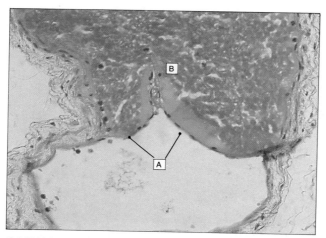

**Q146.** Identify the structures labelled **A** in this vein.

**Q147.** What is their function?

**Q148.** Name a condition in which these structures fail to work?

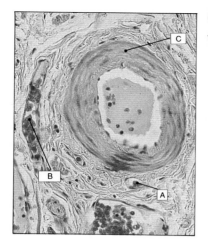

**Q149.** Identify blood vessels **A-C.**

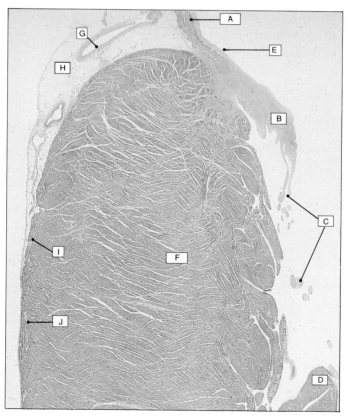

**Q150.** Identify the structures **A-J** in this low power photomicrograph through part of the wall of the left side of the heart.

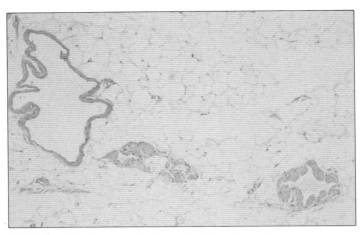

**Q151.** Identify the vessels shown in this micrograph.

**Q152.** What fluid do they contain?

**Q153.** What do they collect the fluid from?

**Q154.** Where do they transport the fluid to?

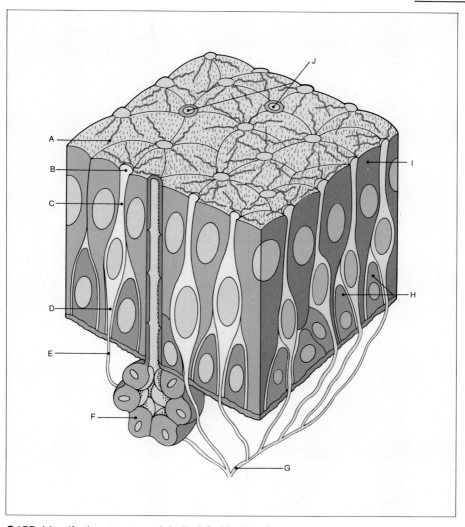

**Q155.** Identify the structures labelled **A-J** in this diagram of the olfactory epithelium from the roof of the nose.

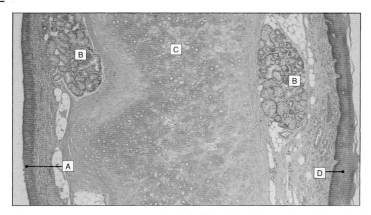

**Q156.** Identify the structures labelled **A-D** in this section through the full thickness of the lower half of the epiglottis.

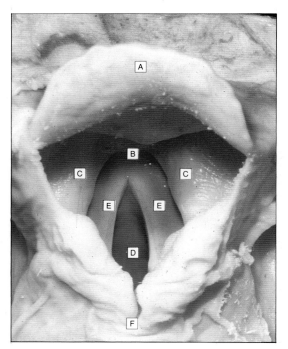

**Q157.** Identify the structures labelled **A-F** in this photograph showing the larynx viewed from above.

**Q158.** Why is structure **B** important in cancer of the true vocal cords?

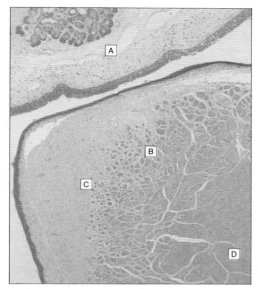

**Q159.** In this micrograph of a vertical section through the larynx the false and true vocal cords are labelled **A** and **B**. Which is which?

**Q160.** What are the differences between **A** and **B**?

**Q161.** Identify the structures **C** and **D** in **B**.

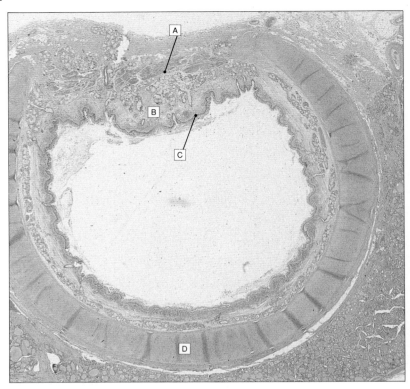

**Q162.** Identify the structure labelled **A-D** in this transverse section of a human trachea.

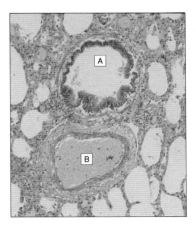

**Q163.** Identify the structures labelled **A** and **B** in this photomicrograph.

**Q164.** Explain why **B** is not a bronchus.

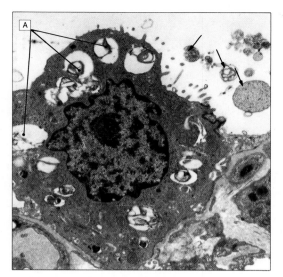

**Q165.** Identify the cell from the alveolar wall shown in this electron micrograph.

**Q166.** What is the function of the bodies labelled **A**?

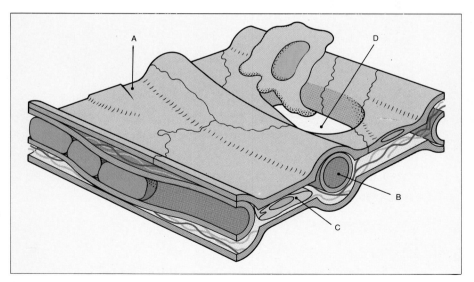

**Q167.** This diagram of the alveolar wall shows (1) pore of Kohn, (2) alveolar wall capillary, (3) type 1 pneumocyte, (4) interalveolar septal macrophage. Match these structures with the labels **A-D**.

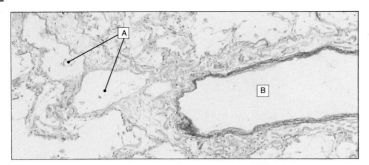

**Q168.** This photomicrograph shows a fibrocollagenous septum in the lung. Identify the structures labelled **A** and **B**.

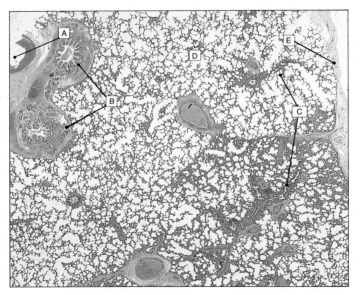

**Q169.** Identify the structures labelled **A-E** in this low power micrograph of the lung.

A = main pi artery
B = branch bronchi
C = bronchiole
D = alveolar
E = visceral pleura

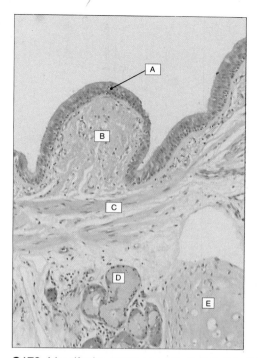

**Q170.** Identify the structures labelled **A-E** in this micrograph of the wall of a bronchus.

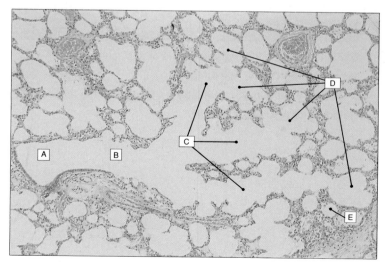

**Q171.** Identify structures **A-E** in this photomicrograph of the distal air passages in longitudinal section.

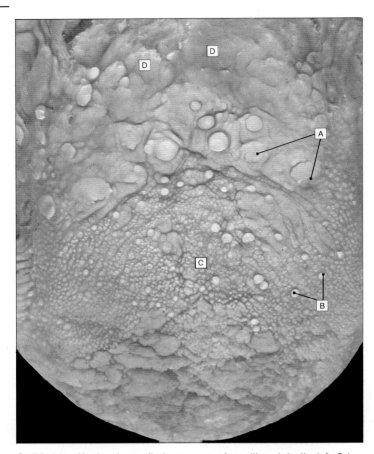

**Q172.** Identify the three distinct types of papillae, labelled **A-C** in this photograph of the human tongue.

**Q173.** What is the pale tissue labelled **D** beneath the mucosa of the posterior third of the tongue?

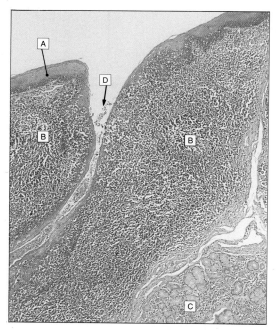

**Q174.** Identify the structures labelled **A-D** in this section from the posterior part of the tongue, showing the lingual tonsillar tissue.

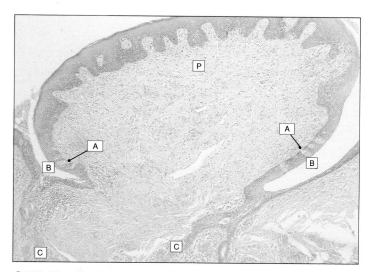

**Q175.** Identify the structures labelled **A-C** in this photomicrograph of a circumvallate papilla (**P**).

**Q176.** What is the function of **A** at this site?

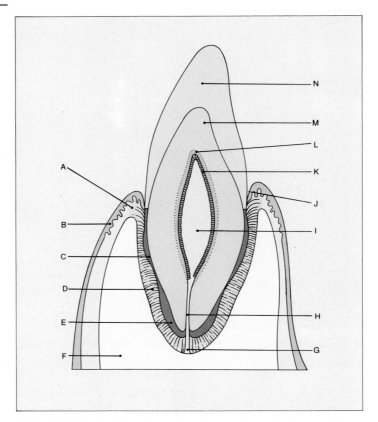

**Q177.** This illustration of a mature human lower incisor tooth shows (1) enamel, (2) dentine, (3) bony socket, (4) periodontal ligament, (5) root canal, (6) pulp cavity, (7) odontoblast layer, (8) gingival epithelium, (9) apical foramen, (10) gingival sulcus, (11) gingival periodontal fibres, (12) cellular cementum (13) acellular cementum, (14) predentine. Match these structures to the labels **A-N**.

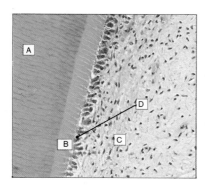

**Q178.** Identify the structures labelled **A-C** in this photomicrograph of human tooth.

**Q179.** What is the cell layer labelled **D**, and what is the function of these cells?

**Q180.** What is responsible for the striated appearance of **A** and **B**?

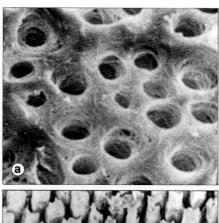

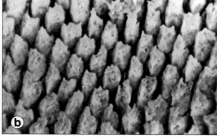

**Q181.** Scanning electron micrographs (a) and (b) shown the mineralized components of mature human tooth. What are they, and which cells produce them?

43

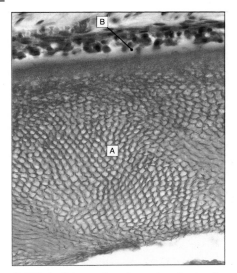

**Q182.** In this section from developing human tooth, identify the material labelled **A** and the degenerating cell layer **B**.

**Q183.** Why is the cell layer degenerating?

**Q184.** What is the basis for the reticulate pattern of **A**?

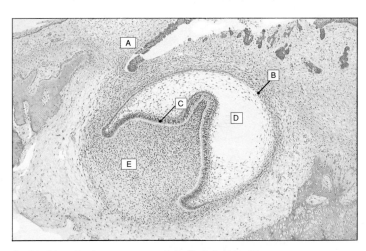

**Q185.** Identify the structures labelled **A-E** in this photomicrograph of a developing tooth.

**Q186.** Which of the structures comprise the enamel organ?

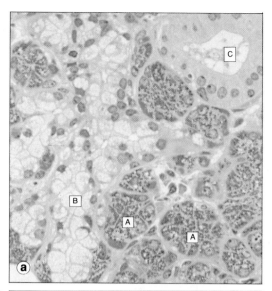

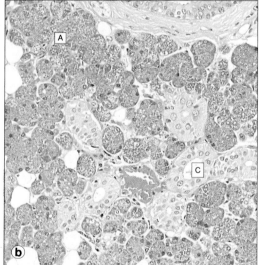

**Q187.** The photomicrographs (a) and (b) show salivary glands of two types - a parotid gland and a submandibular gland. Which is which?

**Q188.** How are the two types distinguished?

**Q189.** Identify the structures labelled **A-C**.

**Q190.** What is the main function of the cells lining **C**, as deduced from their cytoplasmic appearance?

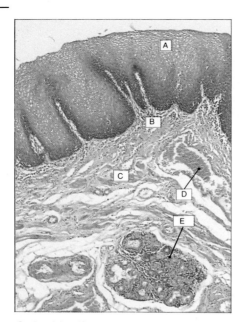

**Q191.** Identify the structures labelled **A-E** in this photo-micrograph of the mucosa and submucosa of the oesophagus.

**Q192.** What abnormality occurs in **C** and **D** in cirrhosis of the liver?

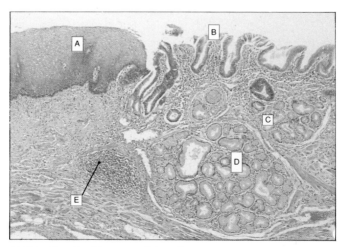

**Q193.** Identify this area of the alimentary tract.

**Q194.** Identify the structures labelled **A-E**.

**Q195.** What is the most common disease that occurs at this site and how does it arise?

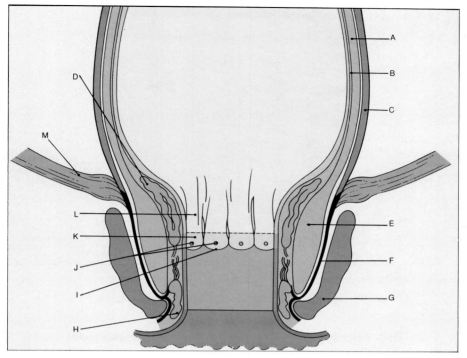

**Q196.** This illustration shows the structure of the anal canal.
Identify the structures labelled **A-M**.

**Q197.** What type of epithelium lines (a) the rectum, (b) the anal canal and (c) the anal skin?

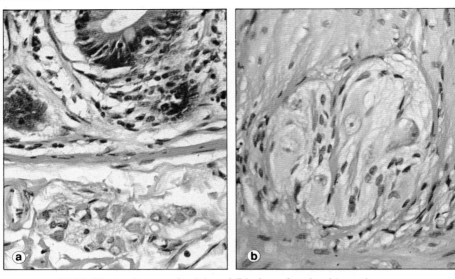

**Q198.** Photomicrographs (a) and (b) show Auerbach's and Meissner's plexuses of nerves and ganglion cells. Which is which?

**Q199.** Which disease results from the absence of ganglion cells in these plexuses in the rectum and colon?

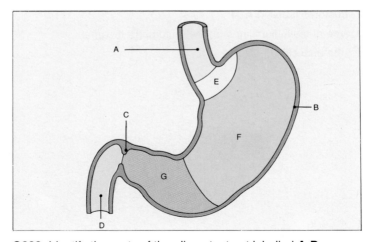

**Q200.** Identify the parts of the alimentry tract labelled **A-D**.

**Q201.** What are the regions of **B** labelled **E**, **F** and **G**, and what is this distinction based on?

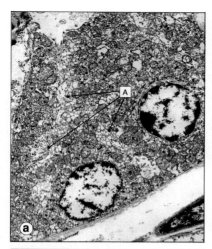

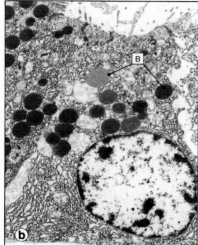

**Q202.** Electron micrographs (a) and (b) show the cytoplasmic features of two of the specialized cells of the glands of the stomach body mucosa. What cell is shown in (a)?

**Q203.** What is its function?

**Q204.** What is the cytoplasmic specialization labelled **A**?

**Q205.** What cell is shown in (b)?

**Q206.** What is its function?

**Q207.** What are the cytoplasmic organelles labelled **B**?

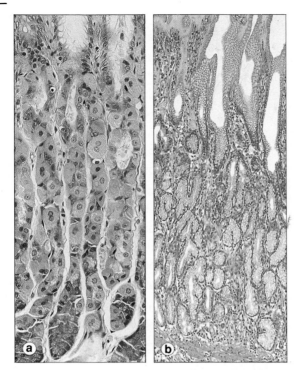

**Q208.** Photomicrographs (a) and (b) show the characteristics of the stomach mucosa from two of the three regions. What are the two regions, and what are the differences in mucosal architecture?

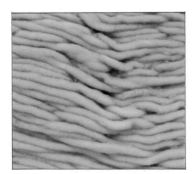

**Q209.** This photograph shows the surface appearance of the mucosa of which part of the alimentary tract?

**Q210.** How is this region identified?

**Q211.** What is the reason for this pattern?

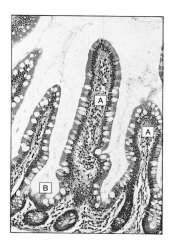

**Q212.** This photomicrograph shows the histology of the mucosa of which part of the alimentary tract?

**Q213.** What are the components labelled **A** and **B**?

**Q214.** What is the purpose of the architectural arrangement of **A**?

**Q215.** What disease is associated with the loss of this architectural arrangement, and what are its consequences?

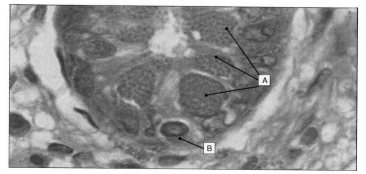

**Q216.** This high magnification photomicrograph shows the base of a gland crypt from the small intestine. Identify the cells labelled **A**.

**Q217.** What do they secrete?

**Q218.** Identify the cell labelled **B**.

**Q219.** What does it secrete?

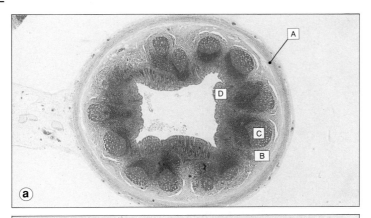

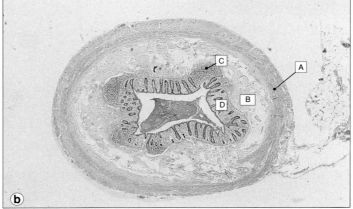

**Q220.** These two photomicrographs shows transverse sections through the human appendix. Identify the structures labelled **A-D.**

**Q221.** One section is from a child, the other from an adult. Which is which?

**Q222.** What distinguishes them?

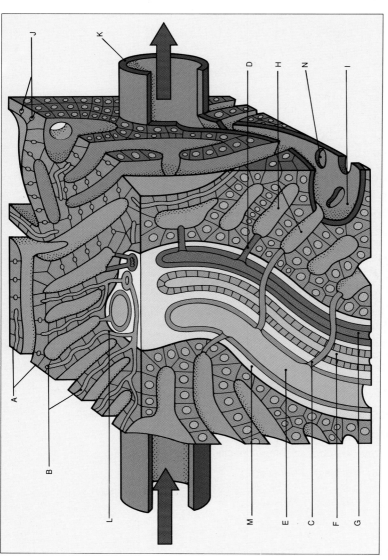

**Q223.** Identify the components labelled **A-N** in this 3-dimensional diagram of liver architecture.

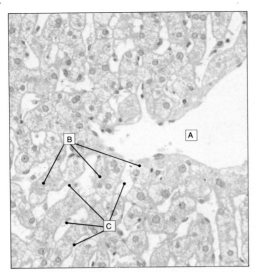

**Q224.** Identify the structures labelled **A-C** in this photomicrograph of liver parenchyma.

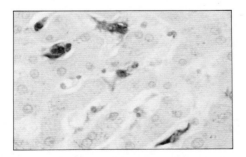

**Q225.** Identify the brown-staining cells located in the sinusoid wall in this photomicrograph of liver, stained by an immunoperoxidase method specific for lysozyme.
**Q226.** What is their function?

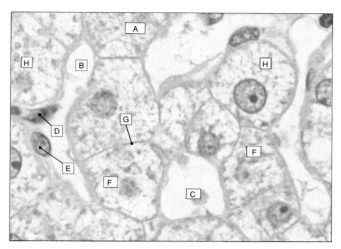

**Q227.** In this high magnification photomicrograph of hepatocytes (**H**), match the following features with the labels **A-G**: (1) sinusoid lumen, (2) sinusoidal surface of hepatocyte, (3) bile canaliculus, (4) canalicular surface of hepatocyte, (5) intercellular surface of hepatocyte, (6) sinusoidal endothelial cell, (7) Kupffer cell.

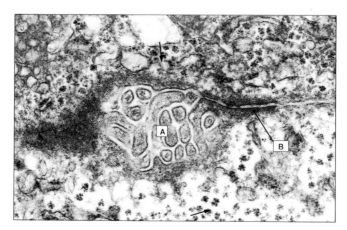

**Q228.** This electron micrograph shows the surfaces of two adjacent hepatocytes. What type of surface is it?

**Q229.** Identify the structures labelled **A** and **B**.

**Q230.** What is the dark granular material (arrowed) in the hepatocyte cytoplasm?

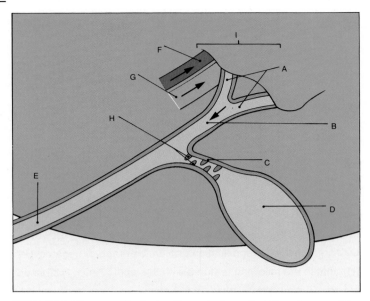

**Q231.** This diagram illustrates the extrahepatic biliary tree and its relationships with the inferior surface of the liver (brown). Identify the components labelled **A-H**.

**Q232.** What are the functions of **D**?

**Q233.** What is the name given to the area **I** where **F** and **G** enter, and **A** emerges from, the liver?

**Q234.** What does **E** drain into?

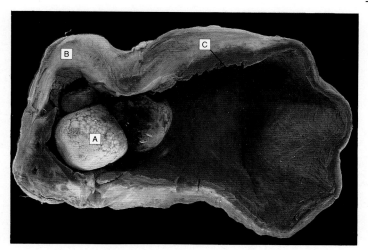

**Q235.** This gross photograph shows a diseased gall bladder.
What are the three main abnormalities, labelled **A-C**?
**Q236.** What is this disease called?

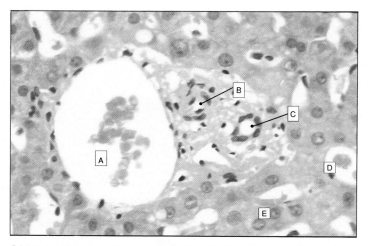

**Q237.** Identify the structures labelled **A-E** in this
photomicrograph of a portal tract in the liver.

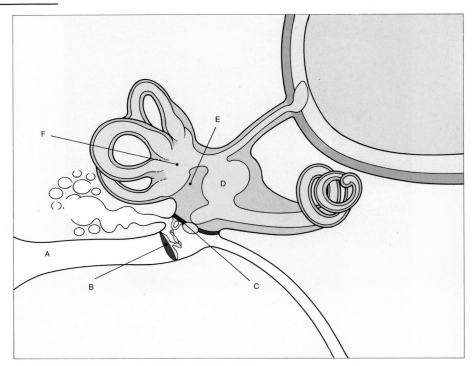

**Q238.** This diagram illustrates the structure of the auditory apparatus. Identify the structures labelled **A-F.**

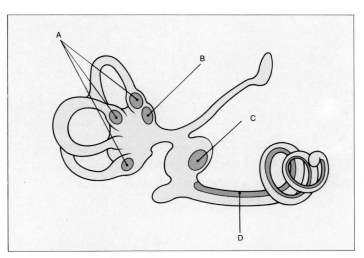

**Q239.** Identify the sensory hair cell-containing structures labelled **A-D** in this diagram of the membranous labyrinth of the ear.

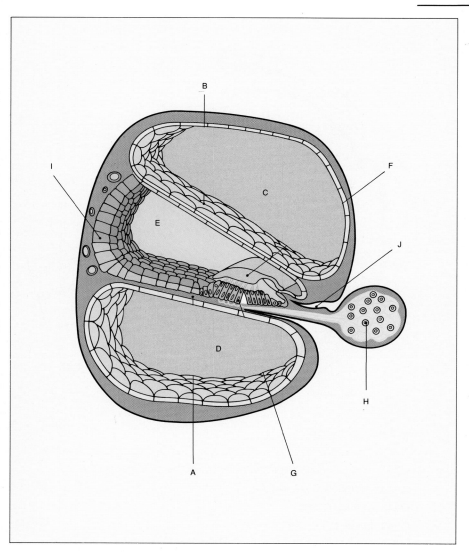

**Q240.** Identify the structures labelled **A-J** in this diagram of a cross-section of the cochlea.

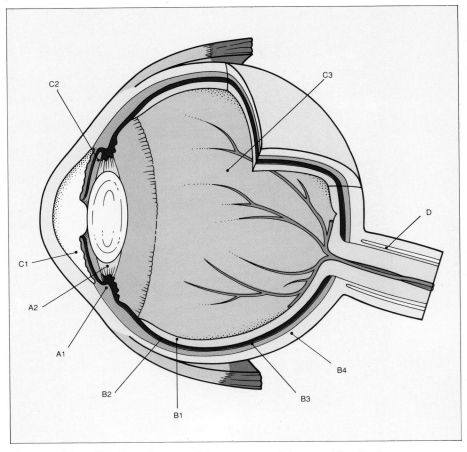

**Q241.** This is a diagram of the anatomy of the eye. Identify the structures labelled **A1** and **A2.**

**Q242.** Identify **B1-B4**.

**Q243.** Identify the cavities **C1-C3**.

**Q244.** What is present in the space of the optic nerve sheath **D**?

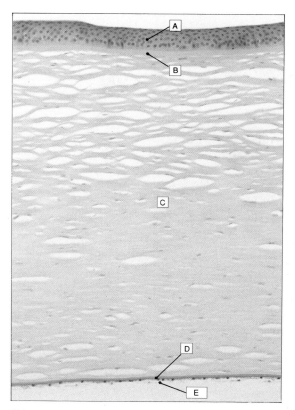

**Q245.** Identify the structures labelled **A-E** in this section of the cornea.

**Q246.** What is the function of layer **E**?

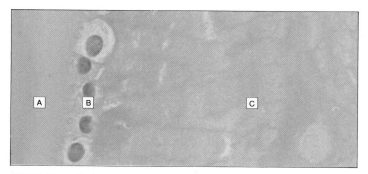

**Q247.** Identify the structures labelled **A-C** in this photomicrograph from the periphery of the lens.

**Q248.** What is the main constituent of structure **C**?

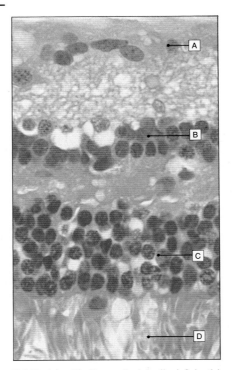

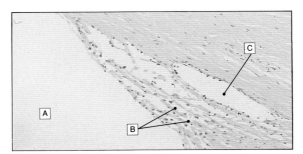

**Q249.** Identify the cells labelled **A** in this photo-micrograph of the retina.

**Q250.** What cells form the inner nuclear layer **B**?

**Q251.** What cells form the outer nuclear layer **C**?

**Q252.** What is found in layer **D**?

**Q253.** Identify the structures labelled **A-C** in this photomicrograph of the eye from the angle between the iris and the cornea.

**Q254.** What is the function of **B** and **C**?

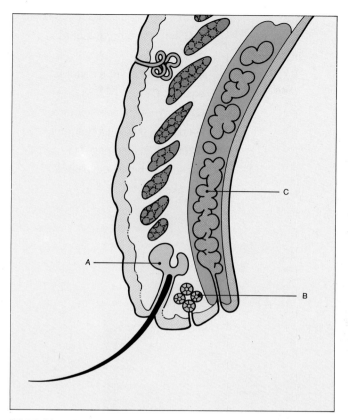

**Q255.** Identify the structures labelled **A-C** in this diagram of the eyelid.

**Q256.** What is the function of **C**?

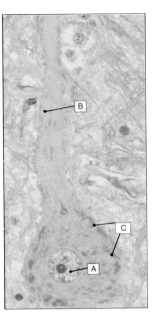

**Q257.** Identify the structures labelled **A-C** in this micrograph of a neuronal cell.

**Q258.** What is the structural basis of **C**?

**Q259.** What class of intermediate filament is present in neurons?

**Q260.** What element of the cytoskeleton is highly developed in the axon?

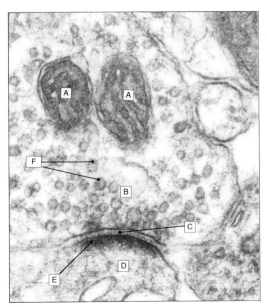

**Q261.** Identify the structures labelled **A-F** in this electronmicrograph of a synapse.

**Q262.** What are the main transmitter substances that cause depolarization of the post-synaptic cell?

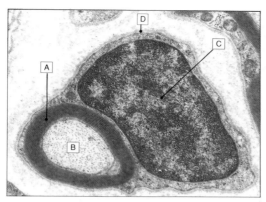

**Q263.** Identify the structures labelled **A-D** in this electronmicrograph from a nerve that has been myelinated in the peripheral nervous system.

**Q264.** What is the function of myelin?

**Q265.** Which cells form myelin in the central nervous system?

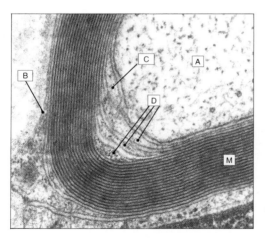

**Q266.** Identify the cytoplasmic areas **B-D** that are associated with myelin (**M**) surrounding an axon (**A**) in this electron micrograph of a portion of myelin sheath.

**Q267.** What is the function of these cytoplasmic areas in myelin?

**Q268.** What is the other main area of cytoplasm in myelin?

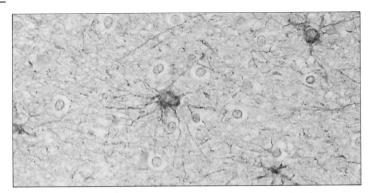

**Q269.** This micrograph shows astrocytes immunostained to reveal their intermediate filament network. What type of intermediate filament is present in these cells?

**Q270.** What function do astrocytes have in embryogenesis?

**Q271.** What function do astrocytes have in the adult central nervous system (CNS)?

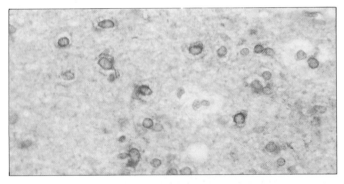

**Q272.** This micrograph shows oligodendrocytes immunostained for a specific oligodendroglial protein. What are the functions of oligodendrocytes?

**Q273.** What histological artefact is useful in the identification of oligodendrocytes?

**Q274.** How does myelination by oligodendrocytes differ from that by Schwann cells?

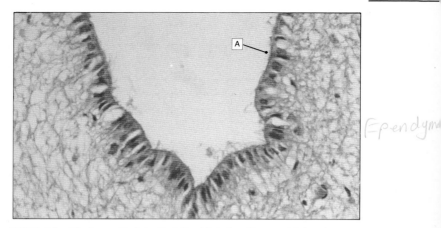

*Ependyma*

**Q275.** Identify the cells labelled **A** which line the ventricle of the brain.

**Q276.** What are the ultrastructural characteristics of this cell type?

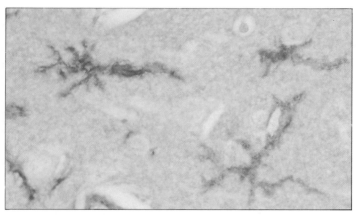

**Q277.** This micrograph shows microglia revealed by immunochemical staining. What is their function?

**Q278.** What is the other main site of macrophagic cells in the CNS?

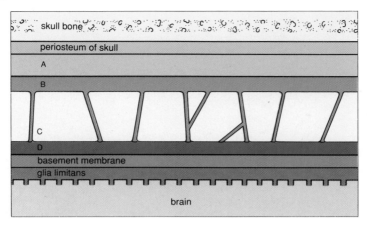

**Q279.** Identify the layers and spaces **A-D** in this diagram of the meninges.

**Q280.** What is present in layer **C**?

**Q281.** In which layer do the blood vessels run to and from the brain?

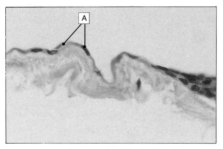

**Q282.** Identify the cells labelled **A** which line the meninges?

**Q283.** What type of cell are these?

**Q284.** What is their main clinical significance?

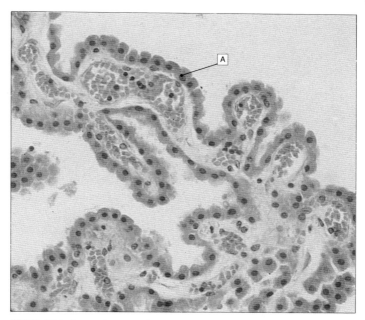

**Q285.** This is a micrograph of choroid plexus. What is its function?

**Q286.** What features of cells **A** adapt them for their function?

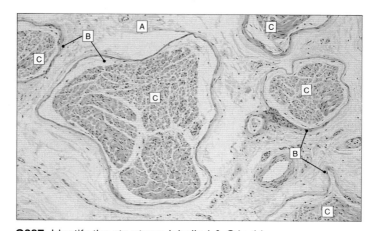

**Q287.** Identify the structures labelled **A-C** in this photomicrograph of a portion of peripheral nerve.

**Q288.** In which area do the main blood vessels of a nerve run?

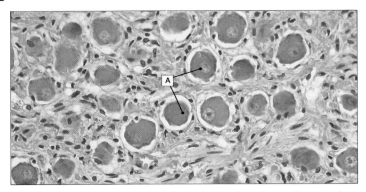

**Q289.** Identify the structures labelled **A** in this photomicrograph of a ganglion.

**Q290.** What other components are present in a ganglion?

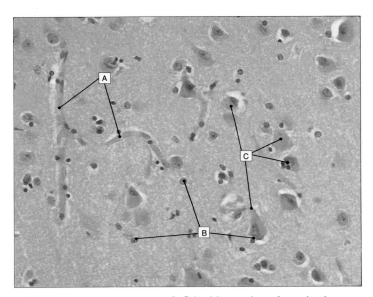

**Q291.** Identify the structures **A-C** in this section of cerebral cortex.

**Q292.** What term is used to describe the pink-staining background of nerve and support cell processes?

**Q293.** Is myelin present in the cerebral cortex?

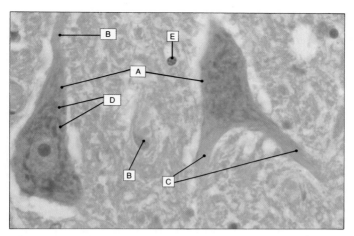

**Q294.** Identify the structures labelled **A-E** in this photomicrograph of neurones from the spinal cord.

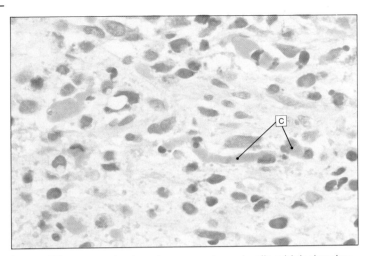

**Q295.** What name is given to mesenchymal cells which develop into skeletal muscle, labelled **C** in this micrograph?

**Q296.** What special name is given to the cell membrane of striated muscle cells?

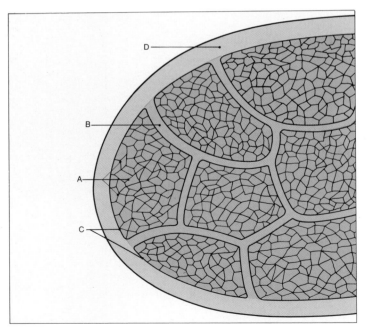

**Q297.** Identify the various components of a muscle, labelled **A-D** in this diagram.

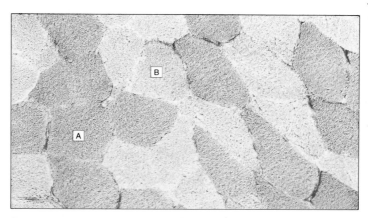

**Q298.** In this micrograph, muscle has been stained by a histochemical method which shows oxidative activity. What name is given to fibres with high activity, labelled **A**?

**Q299.** What name is given to fibres with low activity, labelled **B**?

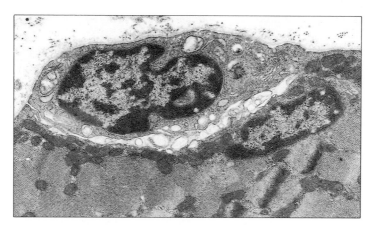

**Q300.** What name is given to the spindle-shaped cell which lies beneath the external lamina of skeletal muscle, as shown in this electronmicrograph?

**Q301.** What is the function of these cells?

**Q302.** What is the normal response of skeletal muscle to increased demand for work?

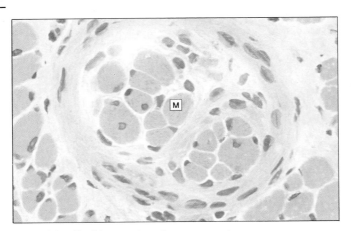

**Q303.** Identify this structure from a muscle.

**Q304.** What is its function?

**Q305.** What two types of intrafusal muscle fibre (**M**) can be identified within this structure?

**Q306.** Describe the innervation of this structure.

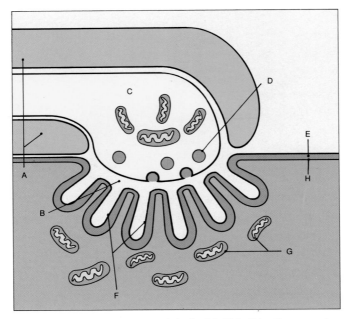

**Q307.** Identify the structures labelled **A-H** in this diagram of a motor end plate.

**Q308.** What transmitter is active in this structure?

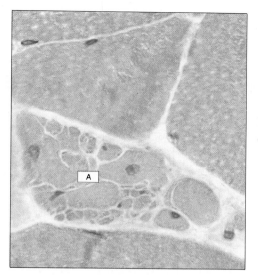

**Q309.** What is the structure labelled **A** in this micrograph of skeletal muscle.

**Q310.** Describe its structural specializations.

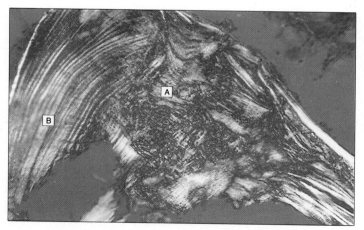

**Q311.** What two types of bone (**A** and **B**) are shown in this polarizing micrograph and how are they distinguished?

**Q312.** What is the main type of bone in the adult?

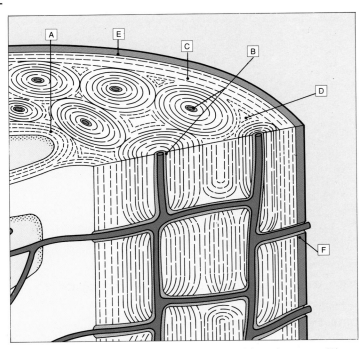

**Q313.** This diagram of cortical bone shows (1) periosteum, (2) haversian canals, (3) inner circumferential lamellae, (4) Volkmann's canal, (5) outer circumferential lamellae, (6) interstitial bone lamellae. Match them with the labels **A-F**.

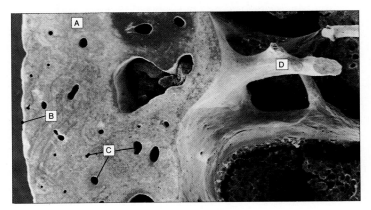

**Q314.** Identify the structures labelled **A-D** in this low power scanning electronmicrograph of a rib bone.

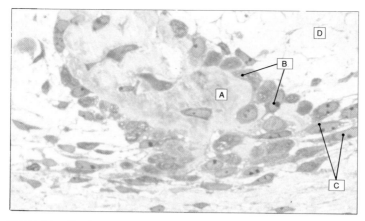

**Q315.** Identify the structures labelled **A-D** in this photomicrograph showing very early bone formation occurring in primitive foetal mesenchyme.

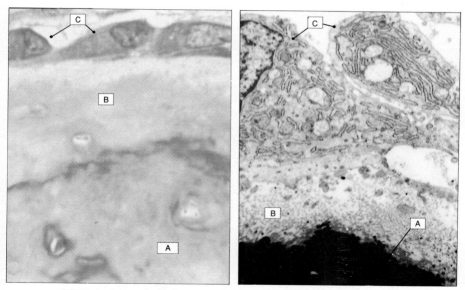

**Q316.** In this paired photomicrograph/electronmicrograph illustration, mineralized bone is labelled **A**. What are the material labelled **B**, and the cells labelled **C**?

**Q317.** What is the most important and prominent cytoplasmic organelle in **C**?

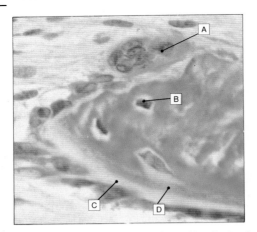

**Q318.** Identify structures **A-D** in this photomicrograph of recently formed bone, stained by a trichrome method whereby fully mineralized bone is stained green.

**Q319.** What are the functions of **A-C**?

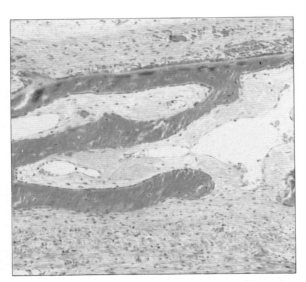

**Q320.** This micrograph shows the pattern of bone formation responsible for the development of the skullbones. What is this process called?

**Q321.** What is the name given to the pattern of bone formation that is mainly involved in the development of the femur and other long bones?

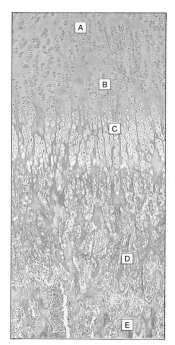

**Q322.** This photomicrograph of the epiphyseal plate region of a lengthening long bone in a growing foetus shows (1) the ossification zone, (2) epiphyseal plate cartilage resting zone, (3) calcified cartilage zone, (4) epiphyseal plate cartilage hypertrophic zone, (5) epiphyseal plate cartilage proliferative zone. Match these zones with those labelled **A-E** in the photomicrograph.

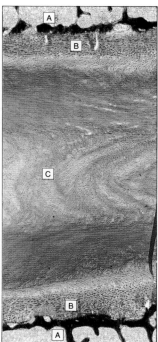

**Q323.** Identify **A**, and the zones labelled **B** and **C**, in this photomicrograph through the full thickness of an intervertebral disc.
**Q324.** What is zone **B** composed of?
**Q325.** What are the two main functions of the intervertebral disc?

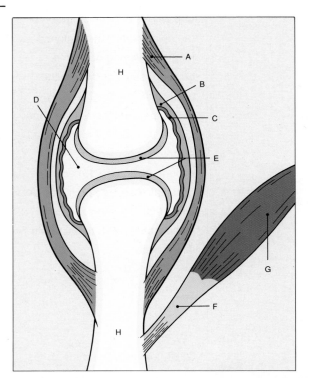

**Q326.** Identify the components labelled **A-H** in this diagram of a typical articular joint.

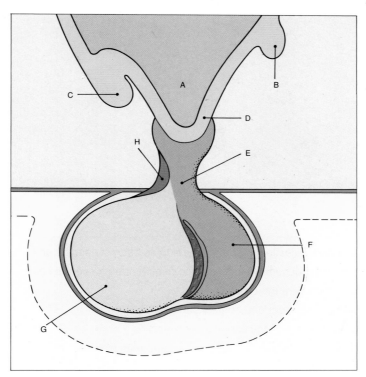

**Q327.** Identify the important components of the pituitary and hypothalamus labelled **A-H** in this diagram.

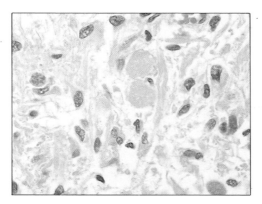

**Q328.** This micrograph is from the pituitary gland. Identify which part.

**Q329.** What hormones are secreted by this part of the pituitary?

**Q330.** What tissues compose this part of the pituitary?

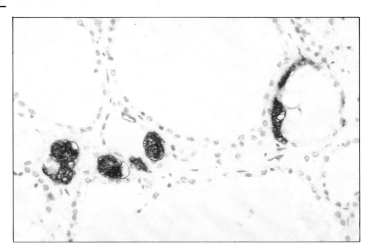

**Q331.** This section of human thyroid has been stained by an immunocytochemical technique to demonstrate a specific cell type. What are the cells?

**Q332.** What hormone do they secrete?

**Q333.** What is the action of the hormone?

**Q334.** What is the ultrastructural appearance of these cells?

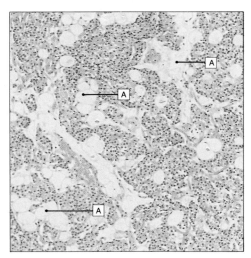

**Q335.** What type of endocrine gland is this?

**Q336.** Which hormone does it secrete?

**Q337.** What is the function of this hormone?

**Q338.** Identify the cells labelled **A**.

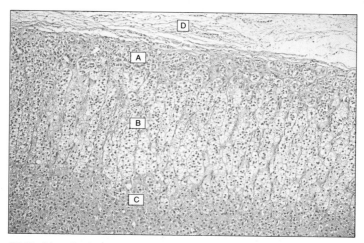

**Q339.** Identify the layers labelled **A-D** in this micrograph of the adrenal gland.

**Q340.** What is the hormone produced by layer **A**?

**Q341.** What is responsible for the pale staining of layer **B**?

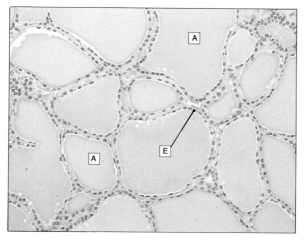

**Q342.** From which endocrine organ is this section taken?

**Q343.** What is the pink material labelled **A**?

**Q344.** What does it contain?

**Q345.** What are the functions of the epithelial cells (**E**) lining the follicles?

**Q346.** What other hormones are produced in this organ, and by what type of cell?

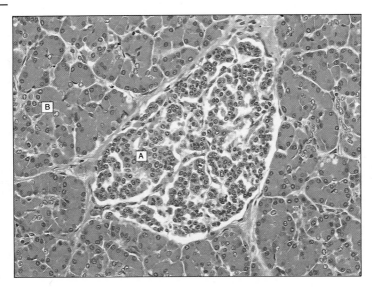

**Q347.** Identify the structure labelled **A**?

**Q348.** What does it produce and secrete?

**Q349.** What is the tissue labelled **B**?

**Q350.** What does it produce and secrete?

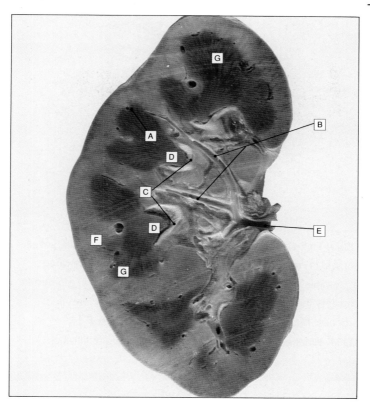

**Q351.** In this gross photograph of a human kidney, the following components can be seen: (1) cortex, (2) medulla, (3) papillae, (4) arcuate vessels, (5) interlobar vessels, (6) main renal artery, (7) calyceal space. Match these structures with the labels **A-G**.

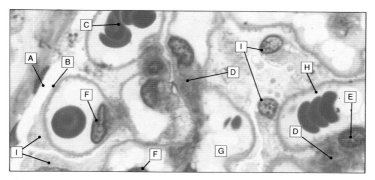

**Q352.** Identify the structures labelled **A-I** in this micrograph of the kidney glomerulus.

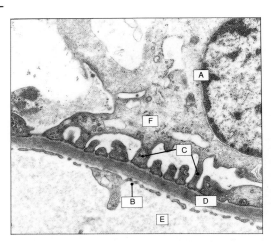

**Q353.** This electron micrograph of the glomerular capillary wall shows: (1) glomerular basement membrane, (2) fenestrated endothelial cell cytoplasm, (3) epithelial podocyte, (4) glomerular capillary lumen, (5) primary foot process, (6) secondary foot process. Match these structures with the labels **A-F**.

**Q354.** What are the components of the glomerular filtration barrier?

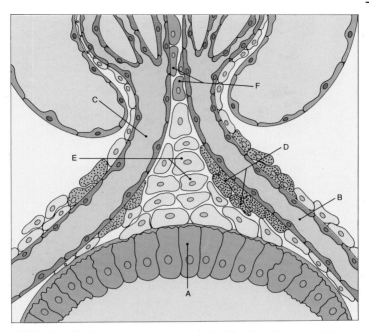

**Q355.** Identify the structures labelled **A-F** in this diagram of the juxtaglomerular apparatus.

**Q356.** What is the role of structure **D**?

**Q357.** In which part of the nephron is structure **A**?

**Q358.** What is the most prominent ultrastructural characteristic of structure **D**?

**Q359.** What is the physiological role of this structure?

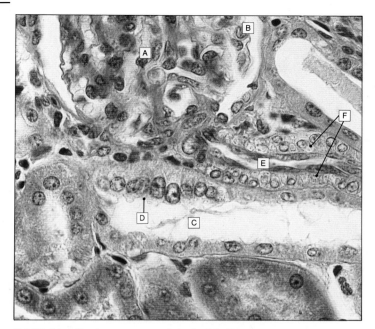

**Q360.** Identify the structures labelled **A-E** in this micrograph of the kidney cortex.

**Q361.** What do the cells labelled **F** produce?

**Q362.** What is the complex comprising **C, D, E** and **F** called?

**Q363.** What other component of the complex is not clearly shown here?

**Q364.** What is the biochemical and physiological function of the substance produced by cells **F**?

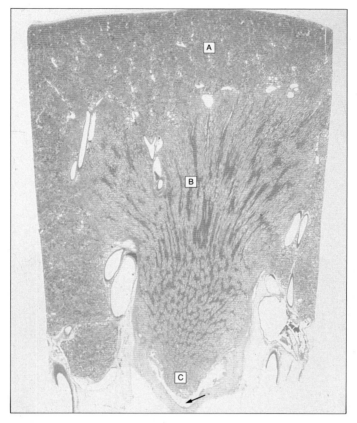

**Q365.** Identify regions **A-C** in this low-power view of the kidney.

**Q366.** What are the red staining, roughly linear streaks in region **B**?

**Q367.** What is the space (arrowed) beyond the tip of **C**?

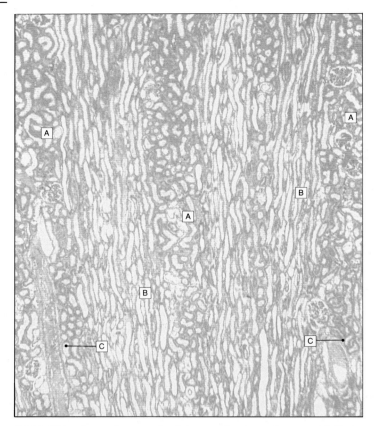

**Q368.** This photomicrograph of the renal cortex shows medullary rays, intralobular arteries and glomeruli-rich zones. Match them with the labels **A-C**.

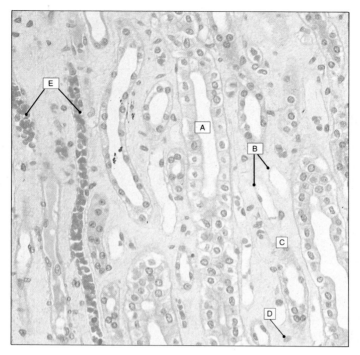

**Q369.** Which part of the kidney is shown here?

**Q370.** Identify the components labelled **A-E**.

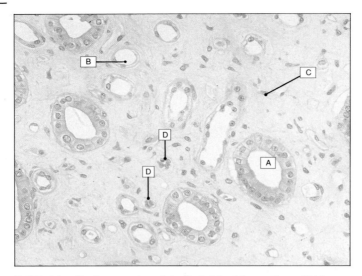

**Q371.** Identify the structure labelled **A** in this section of kidney medulla.

**Q372.** What is its main function?

**Q373.** What is structure **B**?

**Q374.** What is its main function?

**Q375.** What are the cells labelled **C** and the structures labelled **D**?

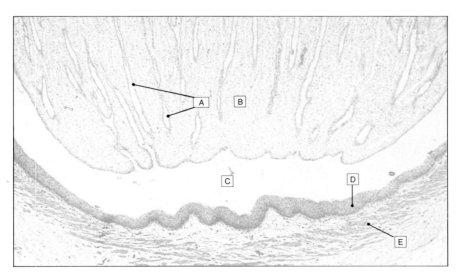

**Q376.** Identify this component of the kidney.

**Q377.** Identify the specific structures labelled **A-E.**

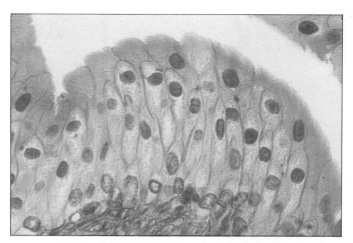

**Q378.** This photomicrograph shows urothelium, the specialized epithelium which lines the lower urinary tract. What are its structural characteristics?

**Q379.** Why does it have this structure?

**Q380.** What specialization does it show on its luminal surface and why?

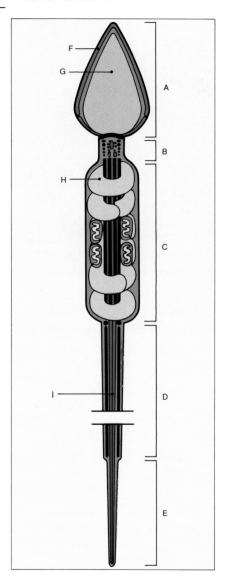

**Q381.** Identify the zones labelled **A-E** and the components labelled **F-I** in this diagram of a mature human spermatozoon.

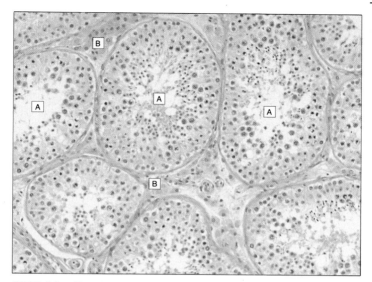

**Q382.** Identify this tissue.

**Q383.** Identify the structures labelled **A** and **B**.

**Q384.** What cells do **A** contain in the mature adult?

**Q385.** What cells do **A** contain in the infant?

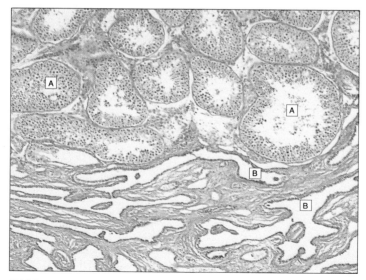

**Q386.** Identify the structures labelled **A** and **B** in this photomicrograph from the hilum of the testis.

**Q387.** Where do the spermatozoa go when they leave **B**?

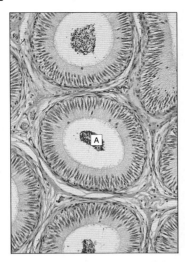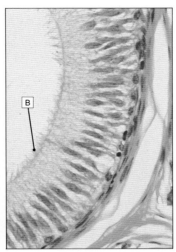

**Q388.** Which component of the male genital system is shown in these micrographs?

**Q389.** What are the structures labelled **A** in the lumina?

**Q390.** What are the structures labelled **B**?

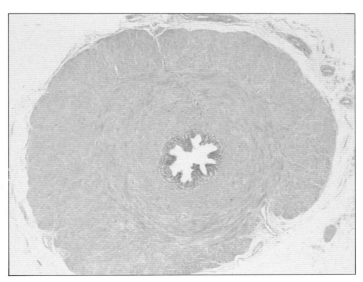

**Q391.** This is a transverse section of a structure in the spermatic cord. Identify the structure.

**Q392.** What is its function?

**Q393.** What else is found in the spermatic cord?

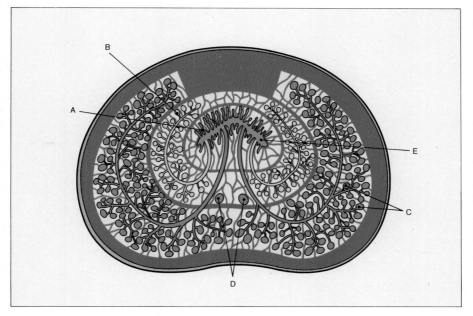

**Q394.** Identify the gland groups labelled **A-C** in this diagram showing their arrangement in a cross-section through the human prostate gland.

**Q395.** Identify the structures labelled **D** and **E**.

**Q396.** What are the two most common and important diseases of this organ, and which gland group does each affect?

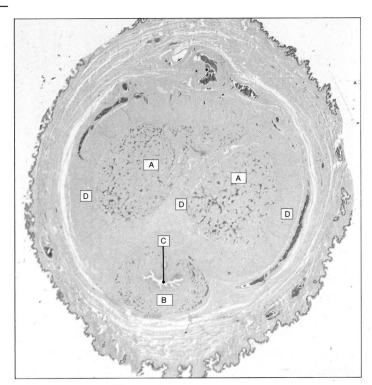

**Q397.** Identify the structures labelled **A-D** in this transverse section through the human penis.

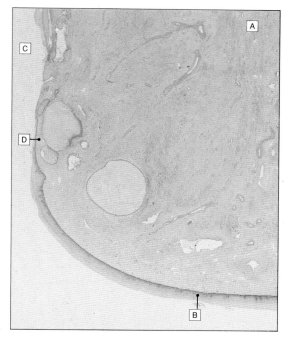

**Q398.** Identify the components labelled **A-D** in this section through the uterine cervix.

**Q399.** What is the importance of the component labelled **D**?

**Q400.** What types of epithelium are present at **C** and **B**?

**Q401.** What cell types make up the bulk of **A**?

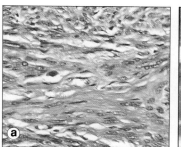 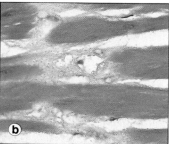

**Q402.** These two photomicrographs show part of the wall of the uterus from two different 26-year-old women. Identify the part shown.

**Q403.** What is the predominant cell type?

**Q404.** How do you account for the difference between the two?

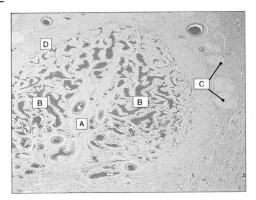

**Q405.** This photomicrograph shows one of the components of the female external genitalia. Identify the structure.

**Q406.** Identify the regions labelled **A-D**.

**Q407.** What type of tissue comprises **B**?

**Q408.** Name two other components of the female external genitalia.

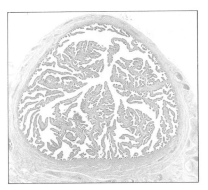

**Q409.** This micrograph shows a transverse section of a component of the female internal genitalia. Identify the component.

**Q410.** Which zone is this component part of?

**Q411.** What is its function?

**Q412.** What are the most important diseases affecting this component?

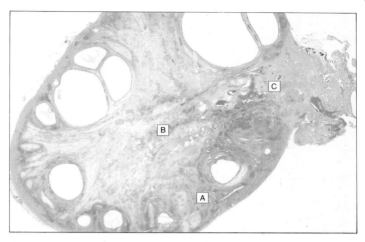

**Q413.** Identify the zones labelled **A-C** in this section through the adult ovary.

**Q414.** What is the origin of the clear cystic spaces in **A**?

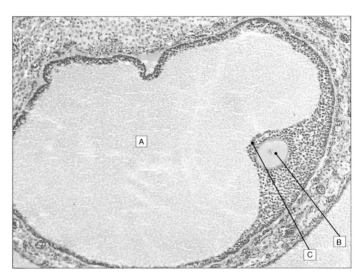

**Q415.** Identify the components labelled **A-C** in this photomicrograph of a mature tertiary follicle in the cortex of the ovary.

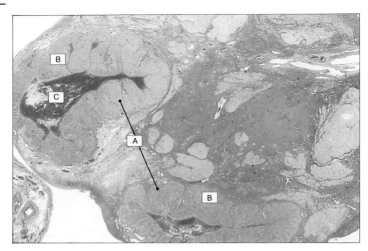

**Q416.** Identify the structures and cells labelled **A-C.** in this micrograph of an adult ovary.

**Q417.** At what stage of the menstrual cycle is the ovary?

**Q418.** How can you tell?

**Q419.** What is unusual about this ovary?

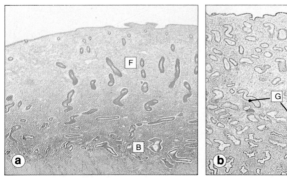
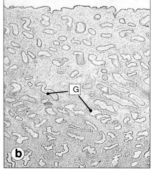

**Q420.** These low power photomicrographs show the endometrial lining of the uterus at various stages of the menstrual cycle, one in the oestrogenic phase (at about 8-10 days) the other in the progesterone phase (at about 18-20 days). Which is which?

**Q421.** What distinguishes the two?

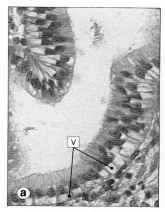

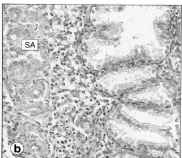

**Q422.** These high power photomicrographs show the endometrial lining of the uterus at two different stages of the menstrual cycle. What stages are they?

**Q423.** What are their distinguishing features?

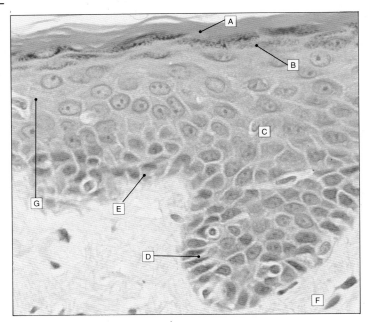

**Q424.** Identify the components labelled **A-F** in this micrograph of a cross-section of human skin.

**Q425.** What is the clear cell labelled **G**?

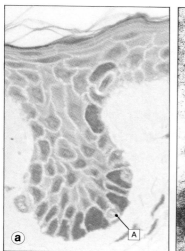
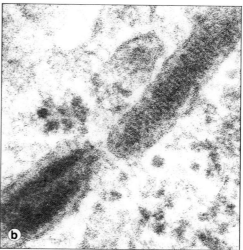

**Q426.** Identify the clear cell labelled **A** in the basal layer of the epidermis.

**Q427.** What is its function?

**Q428.** What is the brown material in the basal cells of the skin?

**Q429.** What are the boat-shaped bodies shown in (b), a high magnification electron micrograph of the clear cell **A**?

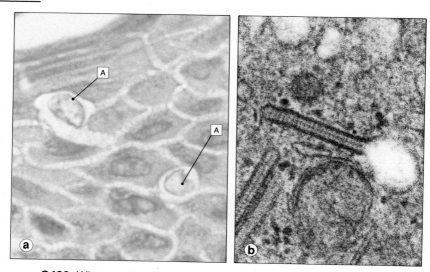

**Q430.** What are the clear cells labelled **A** in this micrograph of the epidermis?

**Q431.** What is their function?

**Q432.** What is the name of their characteristic cytoplasmic organelle shown in high magnification electronmicrograph (b)?

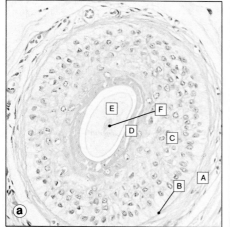 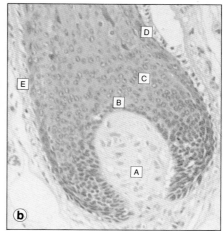

**Q433.** Photomicrograph (a) shows a transverse section of a hair follicle. Identify the components labelled **A-F**.

**Q434.** Is this close to the hair bulb or high up the shaft? Why?

**Q435.** Photomicrograph (b) shows a longitudinal section of the hair bulb or root. Identify the components labelled **A-E**.

**Q436.** Is the patient blonde or brunette? Why?

sebaceous

sweat gland

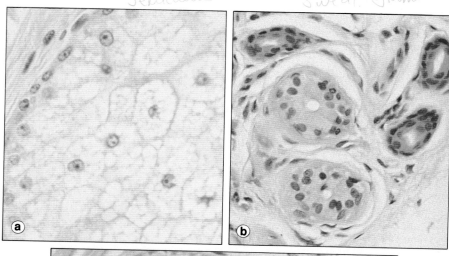

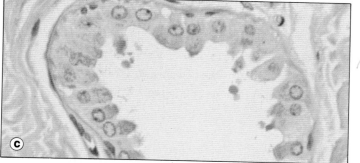

Apo crine

**Q437.** High power photomicrographs (a), (b) and (c) show secretory glands in the skin. Which glands are they, and what does each secrete?

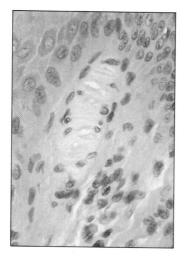

**Q438.** What is this structure, found in the papillary dermis of the skin?

**Q439.** What is its function?

**Q440.** In which areas of skin are they most common?

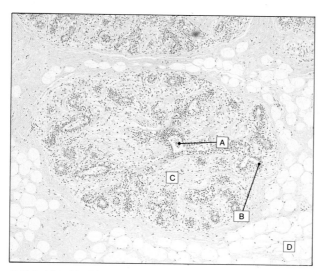

**Q441.** Identify this structure.

**Q442.** In which organ are they found?

**Q443.** Identify the components labelled **A-D.**

**Q444.** Name the two most common and important diseases of this structure.

**A1. A** Euchromatin, **B** Heterochromatin.
**A2.** The nuclear membrane.
**A3.** The nucleolus.
**A4.** Production of ribosomal RNA
see *Histology* p. 12

**A5.** A mitochondrion.
**A6.** Lipid synthesis and fatty acid metabolism.
**A7.** Cristae.
**A8.** Some are manufactured from mitochondrial DNA in the mitochondrion, others from the cell nuclear DNA in the cytoplasm.
see *Histology* p. 13-14

**A9.** The Golgi.
**A10.** Modification of macromolecules by addition of sugars, and of peptides by proteolysis and phosphorylation. Sorting of macromolecules into specific membrane-bound vesicles.
see *Histology* p. 17

**A11.** (a) Golgi vesicles (primary lysosome) bounded by cell membrane with an electron-dense core composed of acid hydrolases; (b) Endolysosomes (secondary lysosomes) Containing acid hydrolases and partly digested material.
**A12.** They are part of the acid vesicle system involved in the degradation of macromolecules within cells.
see *Histology* p. 16-18

**A13.** Microtubules.
**A14.** Tubulin and microtubule-associated proteins (MAPS), which stabilize their structure.
**A15.** Actin (microfilaments) and intermediate filaments.
see *Histology* p. 20

**A16.**    **D** Prophase
        **A** Prometaphase
        **C** Metaphase
        **F** Anaphase
        **E** Telophase
        **B** Cytokinesis
see *Histology* p. 23

**A17.** (a) Simple squamous epithelium; (b) Simple cuboidal epithelium; (c) Simple columnar epithelium.
see *Histology* p. 27

**A18.** Stratified squamous epithelium.
See *Histology* p. 27

**A19.** Pseudostratified columnar epithelium.
**A20.** Cilia.
see *Histology* p. 27

**A21.** Sealing strands.
**A22.** Prevent diffusion of molecules between adjacent cells.
Prevent lateral migration of membrane proteins.
**A23.** Tight junctions.
see *Histology* p. 28-29

**A24.** The actin (microfilaments) in adjacent cells.
**A25.** a actinin and vinculin.
**A26.** Focal contacts, which link the actin filament network
of the cell to the extracellular matrix.
see *Histology* p. 30

**A27.** Intermediate filaments.
**A28.** Adhesion plaques.
**A29.** Desmosomes are a form of anchoring junction. They
provide mechanical stability to cells that are subject to tensile
and shearing stresses, by uniting the intermediate filament
cytoskeleton of adjacent cells.
see *Histology* p. 30

**A30.** Attachment of cells to the extracellular matrix.
**A31.** The intermediate filaments (cytokeratin).
**A32.** Type VII collagen.
see *Histology* p. 31

**A33.** Each junction is a circular patch of membrane studded with
hundreds of pores termed connexons **C**, each formed by six
protein subunits. Pores on adjacent cells are aligned, thereby
allowing free communication between cells.
**A34.** Cells in embryogenesis. Cardiac and smooth muscle.
see *Histology* p. 32

**A35.** A junctional complex.
**A36.** **A** Occluding junction, **B** Adherent junction,
**C** Desmosomal junction.
see *Histology* p. 31

**A37.** Microvilli.

**A38.** Actin, stabilized by actin binding proteins.

**A39.** The cell membrane over the microvilli is associated with enzymes and proteins involved in the absorptive process.

see *Histology* p. 33

**A40.** A cross-section of a cilium.

**A41.** Tubulin.

**A42.** The axoneme.

see *Histology* p. 34

**A43.** Cilia seen in longitudinal section.

**A44.** The basal body from which each cilium arises.

**A45.** The centriole.

see *Histology* p. 34

**A46.** The peripheral microtubules **A** are single and should be double.

**A47.** Failure of clearance of mucus from the respiratory tract; Infertility due to abnormal function of spermatozoa and fallopian tubes; Failure of development of air sinuses in the skull.

see *Histology* p. 35

**A48.** Mucin.

**A49.** Goblet cells.

see *Histology* p. 36

**A50.** Ion-pumping.

**A51.** The basal portion of the cells have a fine striated appearance and are pink staining, This corresponds to the presence of basal folds and mitochondria at the basal surface, which adapt the cell for ion transport and energy production.

see *Histology* p. 37

**A52.** Mesenchyme.

**A53.** Glycosaminoglycans and fibrillar proteins.

see *Histology* p. 42

**A54. A** Elastin, **B** Fibrillin-containing microfibrils.

**A55.** Fibroblasts.

see *Histology* p. 46

**A56.** Overlapping tropocollagen molecules.

**A57.** Reticular fibres are thin fibrils of type III collagen which form a loose supporting framework in tissues, especially lymph nodes, bone marrow and spleen, as well as supporting the basal lamina of cells.

**A58.** Basement membranes.
see *Histology* p. 44

**A59.** Basement membrane.

**A60.** Type IV collagen, laminin, heparan sulphate, entactin, fibronectin, other proteins and glycosaminoglycans.
see *Histology* p. 49

**A61. A** Lamina lucida, **B** Lamina densa,
**C** Fibroreticular lamina
see *Histology* p. 49

**A62.** Cartilage.

**A63.** Type III collagen, glycosaminoglycans (predominantly hyaluronic acid, chondroitin sulphate and keratan sulphate).

**A64.** Chondroblasts.

**A65.** Hyaline cartilage, fibrocartilage, elastic cartilage.
see *Histology* p. 52

**A66.** Unilocular adipose tissue.

**A67.** Capillaries.

**A68.** 1) Energy storage in the form of fat;
2) To act as a deformable shock-absorbing tissue.
see *Histology* p. 54

**A69.** Multilocular adipose tissue.

**A70.** Abundant mitochondria.

**A71.** Generation of heat in the neonatal period.

**A72.** Brown fat.
see *Histology* p. 55

**A73.** Striated (skeletal) muscle.

**A74.** By fusion of myoblasts derived from mesenchyme.

**A75.** Sarcoplasmic membrane, sarcoplasm, sarcoplasmic reticulum.
see *Histology* p. 58

**A76. A** Sarcomere, **B** A band, **C** M line,
**D** Z line, **E** I band, **F** H band.
**A77.** Myosin.
**A78.** Actin.
see *Histology* p. 58

**A79.** Cardiac muscle.
**A80.** Intercalated disc.
**A81.** The intercalated disc is composed of junctional complexes
between adjacent cardiac muscle cells. They have both
anchoring and communicating functions.
see *Histology* p. 63

**A82.** Smooth muscle.
**A83.** An external lamina.
**A84.** By communicating cell junctions, also called nexus junctions.
**A85.** Desmin.
see *Histology* p. 64

**A86.** Bone marrow.
**A87. A** Trabecular bone, **B** Adipose tissue,
**C** Haemopoietic (red) marrow.
see *Histology* p. 67

**A88.** Normal mature red blood cells (erythrocytes).
**A89.** The cells in (c) lack the central pale-staining area
associated with the concave disc shape, shown in (b); the
abnormal cells are spherical (spherocytes).
**A90.** Hereditary spherocytosis due to an inherited defect in the
arrangement of membrane bracing proteins (ankyrin and
spectrin) responsible for maintaining the biconcave disc shape.
see *Histology* p. 68-69

**A91.** Mature neutrophil granulocyte ('polymorph').
**A92.** One, but multilobed.
**A93.** Phagocytosis and destruction of phagocytosed material.
see *Histology* p. 71

**A94. A** Metamyelocyte, **B** Myelocyte, **C** Promyelocyte,
**D** Myeloblast, **E** Stab form.
**A95.** In the haemopoietic bone marrow.
**A96.** Granulocytic, or myeloid, leukaemias
(acute and chronic).
see *Histology* p. 72

**A97.** Eosinophil granulocyte.

**A98.** One, but almost always bilobed.

**A99.** Ovoid or elongated granules containing a central crystalloid.

see *Histology* p. 74

**A100.** Lymphocyte.

**A101.** Antibody production (B lymphocyte) and cell-mediated immunity (T lymphocyte).

see *Histology* p. 75

**A102.** Monocyte.

**A103.** Macrophage/histiocyte.

see *Histology* p. 76

**A104.** Platelets (thrombocytes).

**A105.** Aggregation, to initiate the formation of a thrombus which plugs vessel defects and maintains haemostasis.

**A106.** The platelets are beginning to aggregate, becoming spherical and developing numerous thin cytoplasmic processes.

see *Histology* p. 78

**A107. A** Cortex, **B** Medulla, **C** Septa

**A108.** Epitheliocytes, T cells, macrophages, eosinophils.

**A109.** In much of the thymic cortex, the epitheliocytes are in intimate contact with the lymphocytes, and completely enclose them by deep infoldings of surface membrane. Described as thymic nurse cells, these cells are thought to eliminate immature T cells that recognize self antigens. Epitheliocytes also promote T-cell differentiation, proliferation and subset maturation. In addition, they secrete at least three hormones and other substances, which regulate T-cell maturation and proliferation within the thymus and other lymphoid organs.

see *Histology* p. 87

**A110.** Hassal's corpuscles.

**A111.** Thymic epitheliocytes.

**A112.** The thymic medulla.

see *Histology* p. 87

**A113. A** Afferent lymphatic, **B** Paracortex, **C** Capsule, **D** Sub-capsular sinus, **E** Medullary sinus, **F** Follicle, **G** Medullary cords.

**A114.** B cells.

**A115.** T cells.

**A116.** Through post-capillary venules in the paracortical region.
see *Histology* p. 90

**A117. A** Dark mantle zone; **B** Germinal centre in a
secondary follicle.
**A118. B** lymphocytes, follicular dendritic cells, tingible body
macrophages.
see *Histology* p. 92

**A119.** High endothelial venules.
**A120.** Entry of lymphocytes into the node.
**A121.** Lymphocytes, interdigitating cells, macrophages.
see *Histology* p. 94

**A122. A** Central artery, **B** White pulp, **C** Red pulp.
**A123.** To mount a primary immune response to antigens in the
blood, and to act as a filter to remove aged or abnormal cells
and platelets from the circulation.
see *Histology* p. 96

**A124. A** Sinusoids, **B** Splenic cords.
**A125.** Endothelial cells.
**A126.** The splenic cords consist of a parenchyma, composed of
stellate reticular support cells surrounding a sponge-like network
of cavities, scaffolded by reticulin fibres. Capillaries open into
this parenchyma and allow the entry of blood.
see *Histology* p. 96

**A127.** The sinuses are lined by flat endothelial cells, which rest
on a discontinuous basement membrane interrupted by narrow
slits through which red cells are squeezed. The phagocytic cells
lie adjacent to the sinusoid walls.
**A128.** These phagocytic cells remove red cells and platelets
which become fragmented during passage through the red pulp
and the slits in the sinusoid walls.
see *Histology* p. 96

**A129.** T cells (staining brown) are the class that surround the
central arteries (right). The non-staining B cell area (lower
centre) is a germinal centre located away from the central artery
at the edge of the T cell area.

**A130.** The zone of red pulp surrounding the white pulp (perilymphoid zone) is composed of a series of fine marginal zone sinuses, rich in dendritic antigen presenting cells. This area allows antigens in the blood to be trapped for presentation to the adjacent lymphoid cells.
see *Histology* p. 97

**A131.** The red cells contain small, purple-stained, dot-like inclusions and many are abnormal in shape. There are increased numbers of platelets.
**A132.** Patients who have had a splenectomy do not mount effective immune responses to bacteria circulating in the blood and are prone to development of septicaemia due to *Streptococcus pneumoniae*.
see *Histology* p. 99

**A133. A** Capsule, **B** Subcapsular sinus, **C** Follicles, **D** Cortical sinus.
**A134.** Via the high endothelial venules in the paracortex.
see *Histology* p. 101

**A135. A** Wall of aorta, **B** Coronary ostium, **C** Aortic valve cusp, **D** Commissure between adjacent valve cusps, **E** Wall of left ventricle, **F** Fibrocollagenous valve ring.
**A136.** The coronary ostia **B** mark the origin of the main right and left coronary arteries.
see *Histology* p. 106-107

**A137. A** Lining (endocardium) of left atrium, **B** Valve leaflets, **C** Chordae tendinae, **D** Papillary muscles, **E** Lining of left ventricle.
see *Histology* p. 106-107

**A138. A** Intima, **B** Internal elastic lamina, **C** Smooth muscle of media, **D** External elastic lamina, **E** Collagen of adventitia.
see *Histology* p. 115

**A139. A** Capillary networks, **B** Metarteriole, **C** Venule, **D** Arteriovenous anastomosis.
see *Histology* p. 117

**A140. A** Capillary lumen, **B** Endothelial cell cytoplasm, **C** Capillary basement membrane.
**A141.** Wiebel-Palade bodies.
see *Histology* p. 117

**A142.** Pericytes.

**A143.** They contract and relax to modify the diameter of the vessel lumen.

**A144.** Smooth muscle cells.

see *Histology* p. 118

**A145. A** Intima, **B** Internal elastic lamina, **C** Circumferential smooth muscle of media, **D** Collagen between media and adventitia, **E** Longitudinal smooth muscle of thick adventitia.

see *Histology* p. 118-119

**A146.** Venous valves.

**A147.** To hold blood **B** against gravity and thus prevent it draining back into the peripheral parts of the venous system.

**A148.** Varicose veins in the legs.

see *Histology* p. 123

**A149. A** Capillary, **B** Post-capillary venule.

see *Histology* p. 123

**A150. A** Left atrial wall, **B** Left atrioventricular (mitral) valve, **C** Chordae tendinae, **D** Papillary muscle, **E** Thick endocardium, **F** Myocardium of left ventricle, **G** Branch of coronary artery, **H** Thick pericardium, **I** Medium pericardium, **J** Thin pericardium

see *Histology* p. 122

**A151.** Lymphatic capillaries and venules.

**A152.** Lymph.

**A153.** Tissue spaces.

**A154.** Lymph nodes.

see *Histology* p. 120-121.

**A155.**  **A** Surface cilia
  **B** Olfactory vesicle
  **C** Dendritic process        ⎤ of olfactory receptor cell
  **D** Proximal process
  **E** Non-myelinated axon ⎦

**F** Bowman's gland, **G** Fila olfactoria, **H** Basal cell, **I** Supporting sustacular cell, **J** Opening of Bowman's gland.

see *Histology* p. 126-127

**A156. A** Ciliated pseudostratified columnar epithelium covering the posterior (pharyngo-laryngeal) surface, **B** Sero-mucous secreting glands, **C** Central cartilage plate, **D** Stratified squamous epithelium covering the anterior (lingual) surface.
see *Histology* p. 128

**A157. A** Epiglottis (pharyngo-laryngeal surface), **B** Anterior commissure, **C** False vocal cords, **D** Trachea, **E** True vocal cords, **F** Mucosa of upper oesophagus.
**A158.** The anterior commissure is an area rich in lymphatics and blood vessels, and is therefore a site from which distant tumour spread often originates.
see *Histology* p. 129

**A159. A** False cord, **B** True cord.
**A160.** The false cord contains seromucous secretory glands and is covered by ciliated columnar epithelium; the true cord contains fibres of the vocalis muscle, the vocal ligament, and is covered by stratified squamous epithelium
**A161. C** Vocalis ligament fibres, **D** Vocalis muscle fibres.
see *Histology* p. 129

**A162. A** Trachealis muscle, **B** Submucosal seromucous glands, **C** Ciliated columnar epithelium, **D** Hoop of cartilage.
see *Histology* p. 130

**A163. A** Branch of pulmonary artery, **B** Bronchiole.
**A164. B** is not a bronchus because it contains no cartilage in its wall.
see *Histology* p. 132

**A165.** Type 2 pneumocyte.
**A166.** Synthesis of surfactant substance.
see *Histology* p. 134

**A167. A** 3, **B** 2, **C** 4, **D** 1.
see *Histology* p. 135

**A168. A** Pulmonary lymphatics, **B** Pulmonary vein.
see *Histology* p. 139

**A169. A** Main pulmonary artery, **B** Branch bronchi,
**C** Bronchiole, **D** Alveolar network, **E** Visceral pleura.
see *Histology* p. 141

**A170. A** Ciliated columnar epithelium, **B** Longitudinal bands of
elastin, **C** Circumferential smooth muscle fibres, **D** Bronchial
seromucous glands in submucosa, **E** Part of bronchial cartilage.
see *Histology* p. 130-131, 141

**A171. A** Terminal bronchiole, **B** Respiratory bronchiole,
**C** Alveolar duct, **D** Alveolar sacs, **E** Alveolus.
see *Histology* p. 133, 142.

**A172. A** Circumvallate papillae, **B** Fungiform papillae,
**C** Filiform papillae.

**A173.** Lymphoid tissue, forming the lingual
tonsillar tissue.
see *Histology* p. 144

**A174. A** Surface epithelium (stratified squamous),
**B** Lymphoid tissue, **C** Lingual salivary gland tissue,
**D** Crypt of lingual tonsil.
see *Histology* p. 145

**A175. A** Taste buds, **B** Moat surrounding papilla,
**C** Salivary gland ducts opening into the moat.

**A176.** Perception of bitter taste.
see *Histology* p. 145

**A177. A** 11, **B** 8, **C** 13, **D** 4, **E** 12, **F** 3, **G** 9, **H** 5, **I** 6,
**J** 10, **K** 7, **L** 14, **M** 2, **N** 1.
see *Histology* p. 146-152

**A178. A** Dentine layer, **B** Predentine layer, **C** Pulp cavity.

**A179.** The odontoblast layer. Odontoblasts synthesize and
secrete predentine.

**A180.** Parallel dentinal tubules.
see *Histology* p. 147-148

**A181.** (a) **Dentine**, showing dentinal tubules. Produced by
odontoblasts. (b) **Enamel**, showing tightly packed prisms.
Produced by ameloblasts.
see *Histology* p. 148-149

**A182. A** Enamel, **B** Ameloblast layer.
**A183.** Because enamel formation is complete. Ameloblasts degenerate and never reform, so enamel cannot be replaced.
**A184.** The tightly packed prism structures of the enamel.
see *Histology* p. 149-150

**A185. A** Remnants of dental lamina, **B** External enamel epithelium, **C** Internal enamel epithelium containing ameloblast layer, **D** Central stellate epithelium, **E** Dental papilla.
**A186. B, C** and **D**.
see *Histology* p. 151

**A187.** (a) Submandibular gland, (b) Parotid gland.
**A188.** The submandibular gland has both serous and mucous glands, whereas the parotid gland has only serous glands.
**A189. A** Serous glands, **B** Mucous glands, **C** Striated duct.
**A190.** Ion-pumping.
see *Histology* p. 152-153

**A191. A** Non-keratinizing stratified squamous epithelium,
**B** Lamina propria, **C** Thick and irregular muscularis mucosae,
**D** Prominent submucosal vein, **E** Oesophageal mucous gland.
**A192.** Oesophageal varices - enormously dilated submucosal veins. These vessels are one of the few sites of anastomosis between the hepatic portal venous system and the mainsystemic venous system. In cirrhosis there is a considerable increase in portal venous pressure, leading to distension of the oesophageal vessels by blood trying to escape from the portal venous system.
see *Histology* p. 154, 183

**A193.** The junction between lower oesophagus and upper stomach ('cardia').
**A194. A** Oesophageal stratified squamous epithelium,
**B** Columnar epithelium of superficial zone of stomach mucosa,
**C** Mucous glands of deep zone of stomach mucosa,
**D** Large oesophageal mucous gland cluster at junction,
**E** Lymphoid aggregates.
**A195.** Peptic ulceration, due to reflux of gastric acid and enzymes onto poorly resistant oesophageal squamous epithelium.
see *Histology* p. 155

**A196. A** Circular muscle of rectum, **B** Submucosa, **C** Longitudinal muscle of rectum, **D** Internal haemorrhoidal venous plexus, **E** Internal anal sphincter (a continuation of the circular smooth muscle), **F** Fibro-elastic septum (a continuation of the longitudinal muscle), **G** External anal sphincter (skeletal muscle), **H** External haemorrhoidal venous plexus, **I** Pectinate (dentate) line, **J** Openings of anal glands, **K** Junctional zone of epithelium, **L** Anal column, **M** Muscle of pelvic floor.

**A197.** (a) Tall columnar, (b) non-keratinizing stratified squamous, (c) hair-bearing keratinizing stratified squamous (epidermis).
see *Histology* p. 156-157

**A198.** (a) Meissner's plexus, in the submucosa, (b) Auerbach's plexus, between the circular and longitudinal layers of the muscularis propria.

**A199.** Hirschsprung's disease.
see *Histology* p. 159-160, 173

**A200. A** Oesophagus, **B** Stomach, **C** Pyloric sphincter, **D** Duodenum.,

**A201. E** Cardiac region, **F** Body region and **G** Pyloric region of stomach, based on the different architectural arrangement and cell content of the stomach mucosa.
see *Histology* p. 163-164

**A202.** Oxyntic or parietal (acid-producing) cell.

**A203.** Synthesis and secretion of dilute hydrochloric acid into the gastric lumen.

**A204.** Complex canalicular system.

**A205.** Chief or peptic (enzyme-producing) cell.

**A206.** Synthesis, storage and secretion of pepsinogen, which is con verted into the active proteolytic enzyme pepsin in the gastric lumen.

**A207.** Spherical granules of pepsinogen.
see *Histology* p. 161-162

**A208.** (a) is body region mucosa, (b) is pyloric region mucosa. In the body mucosa, the deep zone consists of long, straight un-branching glands composed of a mixed cell population, mainly acid and enzyme-producing cells. In the pyloric mucosa, the deep zone consists of branched glands, largely composed of mucus secreting cells with only occasional acid- and enzyme-producing cells.
see *Histology* p. 164

**A209.** Small intestine.
**A210.** By the presence of tightly packed
circumferential folds (plicae).
**A211.** To greatly increase the surface area for absorption.
see *Histology* p. 165-167

**A212.** Small intestine,
**A213. A** Villi, **B** Crypts.
**A214.** To greatly increase the surface area for absorption.
**A215.** Coeliac disease, leading to malabsorption of food
see *Histology* p. 165-167

**A216.** Paneth cells.
**A217.** Lysozyme, an antibacterial enzyme.
**A218.** Endocrine cell.
**A219.** Hormones and peptides (serotonin, enteroglucagon,
somatostatin, etc.) which are active locally on the small intestine.
see *Histology* p. 168

**A220. A** Muscle layer, **B** Submucosa, **C** Lymphoid aggregates,
**D** Mucosa.
**A221.** (a) is from a child, (b) is from an adult.
**A222.** In children, the submucosa contains numerous large
lymphoid follicles, and the mucosa contains many lymphocytes
in the lamina propria. This lymphoid component progressively
disappears with increasing age.
see *Histology* p. 172

**A223. A** Hepatocyte cell plates, **B** Bile canaliculi cut
longitudinally, **C** Inlet venule of portal vein branch (E),
**D** Arterio-sinusoidal branch of terminal hepatic artery branch
(G), **E** (see C), **F** Bile ductule, **G** (see D), **H** Sinusoid,
**I** Central terminal hepatic venule ('central vein'),
**J** Bile canaliculi cut transversely, **K** Intercalated (sublobular)
vein, **L** Paraportal bile ductule (Hering), **M** Support tissue,
**N** Sinusoidal openings.
see *Histology* p. 176

**A224. A** Central terminal hepatic venule (central vein),
**B** Hepatocyte cell plates, **C** Sinusoidal spaces between
hepatocyte plates.
see *Histology* p. 178

**A225.** Kupffer cells.
**A226.** Phagocytosis.
see *Histology* p. 178

**A227. A** 5, **B** 1, **C** 2, **D** 7, **E** 6, **F** 3, **G** 4.
see *Histology* p. 179

**A228.** A canalicular surface.
**A229. A** Bile canaliculus, **B** Junctional complex.
**A230.** Clumps of glycogen.
see *Histology* p. 180

**A231. A** Right and left hepatic ducts, **B** Common
hepatic duct, **C** Cyst duct, **D** Gall bladder,
**E** Common bile duct, **F** Hepatic artery entering liver,
**G** Hepatic portal vein entering liver, **H** Spiral valve of Heister.
**A232.** Storage and concentration of bile.
**A233.** Porta hepatis.
**A234.** The duodenum, at the ampulla of Vater.
see *Histology* p. 184

**A235. A** Stone formation, **B** Thickening of gall bladder wall,
**C** Inflammation of lining mucosa, manifest as reddening.
**A236.** Calculous (stone-associated) cholecystitis.
see *Histology* p. 185

**A237. A** Branch of portal vein, **B** Terminal branch of hepatic
artery, **C** Bile ductule, **D** Hepatic sinusoid (containing red blood
cells), **E** Plates of hepatocytes.
see *Histology* p. 186

**A238. A** External auditory canal, **B** Tympanic membrane,
**C** Oval window, **D** Saccule, **E** Vestibule, **F** Utricle
see *Histology* p. 187

**A239. A** Ampullae of semicircular canals, **B** Macula of utricle,
**C** Macula of saccule, **D** Organ of Corti of cochlea.
see *Histology* p. 189

**A240. A** Basilar membrane, **B** Vestibular membrane,
**C** Vestibular cavity, **D** Tympanic cavity, **E** Cochlear duct,
**F** Tectorial membrane, **G** Organ of Corti, **H** Spiral ganglion,
**I** Stria vascularis, **J** Osseous spiral lamina.
see *Histology* p. 190

**A241. A1** Ciliary body, **A2** Suspensory fibres of the lens.
**A242. B1** Retina, **B2** Pigment epithelium, **B3** Choroid,
**B4** Sclera.
**A243. C1** Anterior chamber, **C2** Posterior chamber,
**C3** Vitreous chamber.
**A244.** Cerebrospinal fluid (CSF).
see *Histology* p. 193

**A245. A** Epithelium, **B** Bowman's membrane, **C** Stroma,
**D** Descemet's membrane, **E** Endothelium.
**A246.** The corneal endothelium is composed of ion-pumping
cells which pump fluid from the cornea and maintain its
translucency.
see *Histology* p. 194

**A247. A** Lens capsule, **B** Lens epithelial cells, **C** Lens fibres.
**A248.** The lens fibres are composed of cells that have lost their
nuclei and are packed with transparent proteins termed
'crystallins'.
see *Histology* p. 202

**A249.** Ganglion cells.
**A250.** The inner nuclear layer is made up of the cell bodies of
nerve cells connecting photoreceptors to ganglion cells (i.e.
amacrine cells, bipolar cells, horizontal cells). It also contains cell
bodies of retinal support cells, the Müller cells.
**A251.** Cell bodies of the photoreceptor cells.
**A252.** Rods and cones, the outer and inner segments of the
photoreceptors.
see *Histology* p. 201

**A253. A** Anterior chamber, **B** Trabecular meshwork,
**C** Canal of Schlemm.
**A254.** The aqueous humor in the anterior chamber filters
through the trabecular meshwork and drains via the canal of
Schlemm to venous blood vessels. These structures allow
circulation of the aqueous, to maintain the normal resting
intraocular pressure.
see *Histology* p. 203

**A255. A** Gland of Zeis, **B** Gland of Moll, **C** Meibomian gland.
**A256.** The Meibomian gland secretes a lipid-rich substance
which delays evaporation of the protective tear film.
see *Histology* p. 205

**A257. A** Nucleus, **B** Axon, **C** Nissl substance.
**A258.** Rough endoplasmic reticulum.
**A259.** Neurofilament protein.
**A260.** The microtubule system
see *Histology* p. 206-207

**A261. A** Mitochondria, **B** Synaptic bouton, **C** Synaptic cleft,
**D** Dendrite, **E** Post-synaptic thickening in dendrite, **F** Synaptic
(neurosecreting) vesicles.
**A262.** Acetylcholine and glutamate.
see *Histology* p. 208-209

**A263. A** Myelin sheath, **B** Axon, **C** Schwann cell nucleus,
**D** Basement membrane of Schwann cell.
**A264.** To minimize leakage of current from the axonal
membrane (insulation) and reduce the capacitance of the axon,
both of which increase the speed of nerve conduction.
**A265.** Oligodendrocytes.
see *Histology* p. 211

**A266. B** Outer collar, **C** Inner collar,
**D** Schmidt-Lantermann incisures.
**A267.** They are continuous with the cytoplasm of the cell body
and serve to maintain the cell membrane of the myelin.
**A268.** The paranodal area.
see *Histology* p. 211-212

**A269.** Glial fibrillary acidic protein (GFAP).
**A270.** They guide the migration of developing
neurons in brain growth.
**A271.** • They form a structural scaffolding.
• They act to transport fluid and ions from the
extracellular space.
• They form a physical part of the blood brain barrier.
• They line basement membrane to form a layer around
the CNS called the 'glia limitans'.
see *Histology* p. 213-214, 217

**A272.** The formation of myelin in the CNS, and to act as satellite
cells to neurons in areas of grey matter (cortex and nuclei).
**A273.** A clear 'halo' is seen around the nucleus.
**A274.** A single oligodendrocyte can myelinate several axons
whereas a Schwann cell myelinates only one axon.
see *Histology* p. 214

**A275.** Ependymal cells.

**A276.** Each ependymal cell is linked to adjacent cells by desmosomal junctions. They have surface microvilli and cilia, but do not have a basement membrane.
see *Histology* p. 215

**A277.** The microglia are a form of specialized macrophage with features suggestive of a role as dendritic antigen-presenting cells.
**A278.** Macrophages are present in the perivascular spaces outside the blood-brain barrier.
see *Histology* p. 216

**A279. A** Dura, **B** Arachnoid, **C** Subarachnoid space, **D** Pia.
**A280.** Cerebrospinal fluid (CSF).
**A281. C**, the subarachnoid space.
see *Histology* p. 217

**A282.** Meningothelial cells.
**A283.** Epithelial.
**A284.** They give rise to a common tumour of the nervous system called a 'meningioma'.
see *Histology* p. 217

**A285.** Secretion of the cerebrospinal fluid.
**A286.** The cells are anchored together by junctional complexes (including occluding junctions), have surface microvilli and numerous mitochondria.
see *Histology* p. 218

**A287. A** Epineurium, **B** Perineurium, **C** Nerve fascicles containing axons and endoneurium.
**A288.** In the epineurium.
see *Histology* p. 220

**A289.** Neuronal cells.
**A290.** Support cells (satellite cells and Schwann cells), axons and fibrocollagenous support tissue.
see *Histology* p. 222

**A291. A** Capillaries, **B** Oligodendrocyte nuclei (satellite cells), **C** Neuronal cells.
**A292.** Neuropil.
**A293.** No.
see *Histology* p. 223

**A294. A** Motor neurones, **B** Axon, **C** Dendrites,
**D** Nissl substance, **E** Oligodendrocyte nucleus.
see *Histology* p. 225

**A295.** Rhabdomyoblasts. In embryogenesis, skeletal muscle
develops from mesenchymal tissues with the formation of these
small spindle-shaped mononuclear cells, called rhabdomyoblasts. Multinucleate muscle fibres then form from the fusion
of numerous individual rhabdomyoblasts, and enlarge in size
following connection to the nervous system.
**A296.** Sarcolemma.
see *Histology* p. 226

**A297. A** Endomysium, **B** Perimysium, **C** Muscle fascicles,
**D** Epimysium.
see *Histology* p. 227

**A298.** Type 1 fibres.
**A299.** Type 2 fibres.
see *Histology* p. 228

**A300.** Satellite cell.
**A301.** Satellite cells act as a pool of inactive stem cells in
muscle, which can be stimulated to divide and regenerate
muscle following damage.
**A302.** Normal adult skeletal muscle cells do not undergo cell
division. Any increased demands placed on a muscle, for example
by weight training, result in increased muscle size because the
muscle cells themselves increase in size (i.e. hypertrophy).
see *Histology* p. 229

**A303.** A muscle spindle.
**A304.** The spindle is a specialized sensory organ in muscle
which senses stretch and is involved in the maintenance of
muscle tone.
**A305.** Nuclear bag fibres, with fusiform shape and central
aggregate of nuclei, and nuclear chain fibres with uniform
width and dispersed nuclei.
**A306.** Specialized motor nerve fibres ($\gamma$ efferent fibres) innervate
the intrafusal fibres and adjust their length according to the state of
stretch of the muscle, which is detected by spiral nerve endings.The
spiral nerve endings are wrapped around the intrafusal fibres and
form special sensory afferent fibres running back to the spinal cord.
see *Histology* p. 230

**A307. A** Schwann cell, **B** Synaptic cleft, **C** Axon terminal,
**D** Secretory granule, **E** External lamina, **F** Junctional folds,
**G** Skeletal muscle mitochondria, **H** Muscle cell membrane.
**A308.** Acetylcholine.
see *Histology* p. 231

**A309.** A myotendinous junction.
**A310.** At the point where skeletal muscle is attached to a tendon
(or fascia) individual skeletal muscle fibres develop a complex
interdigitating surface, which is tightly anchoredto the support
tissues. This micrograph of a myotendinous junctionshows
apparent splitting of the rounded contour of a muscle fibre to form
several small rounded structures, separated by fibrocollagenous
tissue. Such splitting of the terminal portion of the fibre increases
the surface area available for anchorage to support tissues, and
thus contributes to the mechanical strength of insertion.
see *Histology* p. 232

**A311.** Two types of bone can be identified according to the
pattern of collagen forming the osteoid: **woven bone (A)** is
characterized by haphazard organization of collagen fibres and
is mechanically weak; **lamellar bone (B)** is characterized by
regular parallel alignment of collagen into sheets (lamellae), and
is mechanically strong.
**A312.** Lamellar bone.
see *Histology* p. 233

**A313. A** 3, **B** 2, **C** 5, **D** 6, **E** 1, **F** 4.
see *Histology* p. 234

**A314. A** Cortical bone, **B** Periosteum, **C** Haversian canal
systems, **D** Trabecular bone,
see *Histology* p. 234

**A315. A** Osteoid, recently synthesized by **B** Osteoblasts,
derived from **C** Osteoprogenitor cells, derived from
**D** Primitive mesenchyme.
see *Histology* p. 235

**A316. B** Recently synthesized, as yet unmineralized, osteoid;
**C** Osteoblasts actively synthesizing osteoid.
**A317.** Abundant rough endoplasmic reticulum, responsible for
the synthesis of osteoid collagen.
see *Histology* p. 236

**A318. A** Osteoclast, **B** Osteocyte, **C** Osteoblast,
**D** Recently formed osteoid.
**A319.** Osteoclast - resorption of mineralized bone in
remodelling;
Osteocyte - presumed to be nutrition of bone;
Osteoblast - synthesis of osteoid collagen,
see *Histology* p. 238

**A320.** Intramembranous ossification.
**A321.** Endochondral ossification.
see *Histology* p. 243

**A322. A** 2, **B** 5, **C** 4, **D** 3, **E** 1.
see *Histology* p. 245

**A323. A** Parts of adjacent vertebral bodies,
**B** Annulus fibrosus, **C** Nucleus pulposus.
**A324.** Fibrocartilage.
**A325.** Functions as a shock-absorber and also
permits limited flexion and extension of the spine.
see *Histology* p. 246

**A326. A** Ligament, **B** Fibrous joint capsule, **C** Synovium,
**D** Synovial cavity (joint space), **E** Articular cartilage covering
bone ends, **F** Tendon, whereby **G** Skeletal muscle attaches
to bone, **H** Long bones.
see *Histology* p. 247

**A327. A** Cavity of third ventricle of the brain, **B** Mamillary body of
the brain, **C** Optic chiasm, **D** Median eminence of hypothalamus,
**E** Pituitary stalk of posterior pituitary (neurohypophysis),
**F** Neural lobe of posterior pituitary (neurohypophysis),
**G** Distal lobe of anterior pituitary (adenohypophysis),
**H** Tuberal lobe of anterior pituitary (adenohypophysis).
see *Histology* p. 250

**A328.** The posterior (neural) pituitary.
**A329.** Oxytocin and antidiuretic hormone.
**A330.** Axons derived from neuronal cells in the
hypothalamus and glial cells termed 'pituicytes'.
see *Histology* p. 254

**A331.** C cells.
**A332.** Calcitonin.

**A333.** Inhibits the resorption of calcium from bone byosteoclasts.
**A334.** Neuroendocrine cells containing dense-core neurosecretory granules.
see *Histology* p. 258

**A335.** The parathyroid gland.
**A336.** Parathormone.
**A337.** It is central to calcium metabolism and is secreted by the gland in response to hypocalcaemia, causing stimulation of osteoclasts to release calcium from bone.
**A338.** Adipocytes.
see *Histology* p. 259

**A339. A** Zona glomerulosa, **B** Zona fasciculata, **C** Zona reticularis, **D** Capsule.
**A340.** Aldosterone.
**A341.** The cells of the zona fasciculata contain abundant cholesterol lipid which is removed in tissue processing to leave pale-stained cells.
see *Histology* p. 261

**A342.** Thyroid gland.
**A343.** Thyroid colloid.
**A344.** Iodinated thyroglobulin in storage form.
**A345.** Synthesis of thyroglobulin and transfer into follicle lumen; Transport of iodine into colloid in follicle lumen; Reabsorption of stored iodinated thyroglobulin; Breakdown of iodinated thyroglobulin into active thyroid hormone (thyroxine); Secretion of thyroxine into blood stream.
**A346.** Calcitonin, by the thyroid C cells.
see *Histology* p. 257-258, 269

**A347.** Islet of Langerhans.
**A348.** Hormones, including insulin, amylin, glucagon, pancreatic polypeptide and somatostatin.
**A349.** Exocrine pancreatic tissue.
**A350.** Enzymes involved in the digestion of food in the alimentary tract, including amylase, lipase and trypsinogen.
see *Histology* p. 169, 264.

**A351. A** 4, **B** 5, **C** 7, **D** 3, **E** 6, **F** 1, **G** 2.
see *Histology* p. 272

**A352. A** Epithelial cells lining Bowman's capsule, **B** Urinary (Bowman's) space, **C** Red blood cells in glomerular capillary lumen, **D** Mesangium (matrix), **E** Mesangium (cell nucleus), **F** Nucleus of endothelial cell lining interior of glomerular capillary lumen, **G** Glomerular capillary lumen, **H** Glomerular capillary basement membrane, **I** Epithelial cell (podocyte) covering outer surface of glomerular capillary.
see *Histology* p. 277

**A353. A** 3, **B** 2, **C** 6, **D** 1, **E** 4, **F** 5.

**A354.** The glomerular filtration barrier is composed of:
- the capillary endothelial inner layer (**B**);
- the unusually thick glomerular capillary basement membrane (**D**);
- the podocyte (the outer epithelial layer) (**A**).

see *Histology* p. 278

**A355. A** Macula densa, **B** Afferent arteriole, **C** Efferent arteriole, **D** Granular cells, **E** Lacis cells, **F** Glomerular mesangial cells.

**A356.** Secretion of renin.

**A357.** In the distal tubule, close to the junction between the straight and convoluted parts.

**A358.** Contractile filaments and neuroendocrine granules.

**A359.** Renin secreted by the juxtaglomerular apparatus causes sodium and water retention by the kidney. This structure is therefore important for blood pressure regulation and electrolyte and fluid balance.
see *Histology* p. 293

**A360. A** Glomerulus, **B** Urinary (Bowman's) space, **C** Distal tubule (lumen), **D** Cells of macula densa, **E** Afferent arteriole (lumen).

**A361.** Renin.

**A362.** The juxtaglomerular apparatus.

**A363.** Lacis cells.

**A364.** Renin catalyses the production of angiotensin I from its inactive precursor, angiotensinogen. Angiotensin I is converted into the active octapeptide angiotensin II in the lung. Angiotensin II then stimulates the release of aldosterone from the adrenal cortex. Aldosterone mediates the absorption of sodium and water from the glomerular filtrate at the distal tubule, thus maintaining plasma volume and blood pressure.
see *Histology* p. 293

**A365. A** Cortex, **B** Medulla, **C** Papilla.

**A366.** Clusters of vertically running blood vessels, the vasa recta.

**A367.** The calyx.

see *Histology* p. 296

**A368. A** Glomeruli-rich zones, **B** Medullary ray, **C** Interlobular artery.

see *Histology* p. 295

**A369.** Renal medulla (in longitudinal section).

**A370. A** Collecting duct, **B** Thin loop of Henle, **C** Medullary
interstitium, **D** Medullary interstitial cells, **E** Vasa recta.

see *Histology* p. 298

**A371.** Medullary collecting duct.

**A372.** Reabsorption of water from dilute urine under the influence
of anti-diuretic hormone.

**A373.** Thin loop of Henle.

**A374.** Differential movement of water and ions.

**A375. C** Medullary interstitial cells, **D** Thin-walled capillaries.

see *Histology* p. 299

**A376.** A renal papilla, the pointed tip of the medulla.

**A377. A** Collecting ducts at papillary tip (papillary ducts of Bellini),
**B** Medullary interstitium, **C** Calyceal lumen,
**D** Urothelium lining calyx, **E** Smooth muscle of calyx wall.

see *Histology* p. 299

**A378.** Multilayered, compact cuboidal basal layer, and tall
columnar upper layers, often containing binucleate cells.
It has a 'fuzzy' luminal surface.

**A379.** To allow for maintenance of the lining when the lower
urinary tract is distended with urine. The cells flatten and
form a thinner layer.

**A380.** The luminal surface membrane bears rigid invaginations
('membrane plaques') which are continous with membrane-lined
multilaminate vesicles. These provide a reservoir of cell membrane
material that can be quickly incorporated into the luminal surface
when the cells are flattened and stretched during distension.

see *Histology* p. 301

**A381. A** Head, **B** Neck, **C** Middle piece, **D** Principle piece, **E** End
piece, **F** Acrosomal cap, **G** Nucleus, **H** Spiral mitochondria,
**I** Axoneme.

see *Histology* p. 310

**A382.** Mature adult testis.

**A383. A** Seminiferous tubules, **B** Clusters of interstitial (Leydig) cells.

**A384.** Sertoli cells, plus germinal (seminiferous) cells maturing to spermatozoa.

**A385.** Sertoli cells only.

see *Histology* p. 307

**A386. A** Seminiferous tubules, **B** Channels of rete testis network.

**A387.** Into the efferent ductules, and thence into the epididymal duct.

see *Histology* p. 312

**A388.** Epididymal duct.

**A389.** Spermatozoa.

**A390.** Extremely long microvilli (**not** cilia).

see *Histology* p. 313

**A391.** Ductus (vas) deferens.

**A392.** Transport of motile spermatozoa from the epididymis to the ejaculatory duct.

**A393.** Testicular artery, pampiniform plexus of veins, nerves, lymphatic vessels and adipose tissue.

see *Histology* p. 314

**A394. A** Inner periurethral (mucosal) glands, **B** Outer periurethral (submucosal) glands, **C** Peripheral zone (true prostatic) glands.

**A395. D** Right and left ejaculatory ducts passing through prostate before entering the urethra, **E** Urethra passing through prostate after leaving bladder and before entering penis (prostatic urethra).

**A396.** Benign prostatic hyperplasia (affects gland groups **A** and **B**, but mainly **B**), and carcinoma of the prostate (affects gland group **C**).

see *Histology* p. 315

**A397. A** Corpora cavernosa, **B** Corpus spongiosum, **C** Urethra (penile), **D** Fibrocollagenous capsule.

see *Histology* p. 318

**A398. A** Cervical stroma, **B** Ectocervix, **C** Endocervical canal, **D** Transitional zone of epithelium.

**A399.** The transitional zone is the most common
site for the development of cancer of the cervix.

**A400.** The endocervical canal (**C**) is lined by tall columnar
mucus-secreting epithelium. The ectocervix (**B**) is covered by
non-keratinizing, stratified squamous epithelium.

**A401.** Support cells (fibroblasts producing collagen) and
contractile cells (smooth muscle cells).
see *Histology* p. 326

**A402.** Myometrium.

**A403.** Smooth muscle cells.

**A404.** The woman whose myometrium is shown
in (b) is pregnant; the smooth muscle cells are greatly
increased in size thereby increasing the contractile
capability of the uterine wall.
see *Histology* p. 329

**A405.** The clitoris

**A406. A** Central septum, **B** Corpora cavernosa, **C** Pacinian
touch corpuscles, **D** Fibrocollagenous sheath.

**A407.** The corpora cavernosa are composed of
interconnecting vascular channels, which can be
engorged with blood, thus producing erectile tissue.

**A408.** Labia majora and labia minora.
see *Histology* p. 323

**A409.** Fallopian tube.

**A410.** Ampullary zone.

**A411.** Conduction of the unfertilized ovum from the ovary to the
body of the uterus. Fertilization may also occur here.

**A412.** Infection (acute salpingitis), and occasional
implantation of fertilized ovum (tubal ectopic pregnancy).
see *Histology* p. 331-332, 343

**A413. A** Cortex, **B** Medulla, **C** Hilum.

**A414.** The cysts are a mixture of germinal inclusion cysts and
follicular cysts, derived from effete ovarian follicles.
see *Histology* p. 333

**A415. A** Fluid-filled antrum, **B** Oocyte, **C** Cumulus oophorus of
granulosa cells enclosing the oocyte.
see *Histology* p. 337

**A416. A** Corpora lutea, **B** Granulosa lutein cells,
**C** Central blood clot.
**A417.** This ovary is in the progesterone or 'secretory' phase
(day 15-25).
**A418.** The ovarian tertiary follicles have ruptured (about day 15)
and converted into corpora lutea.
**A419.** Two tertiary follicles have ripened and ruptured in this
ovary, with the release of two oocytes. This could potentially
produce non-identical twins or, if the other ovary has also
produced a mature ovum, even triplets!
see *Histology* p. 338

**A420.** (a) is in the oestrogenic phase, (b) is in the progesterone
phase.
**A421.** In (a) the glands of the endometrial layer (**F**) are
proliferating from the compact basal layer (**B**). They are scanty,
tubular and devoid of secretion. In (b) the glands (**G**) are bulky,
tortuous, and filled with secretion.
see *Histology* p. 341

**A422.** (a) is at about day 15-16, i.e. at the time of ovulation,
indicating abrupt transition between the oestrogenic
(proliferative) and progesterone (secretory) phase;
(b) is at about day 25-27, i.e. premenstrual.
**A423.** In (a) the presence of subnuclear vacuolation (**V**)
indicates that ovulation has taken place, and is the earliest sign
of secretory activity. In (b) the convoluted distended endometrial
glands on the right indicate that the endometrium is in the late
secretory phase, and the twisting of the thick-walled spiral
arterioles (**SA**) indicates that menstrual endometrial necrosis and
shedding are imminent.
see *Histology* p. 341

**A424. A** Acellular layer of keratin flakes, **B** Granular keratinocyte
layer containing keratohyaline, **C** Prickle cell layer of
keratinocytes, **D** Basal layer of keratinocytes, **E** Basement
membrane at dermo-epidermal junction, **F** Papillary dermis.
**A425.** Langerhans' cell.
see *Histology* p. 349

**A426.** Melanocyte.
**A427.** Synthesis of melanin pigment and transport
into keratinocytes.

**A428.** Melanin pigment.
**A429.** Premelanosomes.
see *Histology* p. 353

**A430.** Langerhans' cells.
**A431.** Antigen recognition.
**A432.** Birbeck granules.
see *Histology* p. 354

**A433. A** Fibrocollagenous root sheath, **B** Glassy membrane,
forming outer limits of: **C** cells of external root sheath,
**D** Degenerating internal root sheath, **E** Hair shaft,
**F** Central medullary remnant.
**A434.** High, because the hair shaft is devoid of nuclei and the
internal root sheath is degenerate.
**A435. A** Dermal hair papilla; precursor cells of **B** Hair medulla,
**C** Hair cortex and **D** Hair cuticle, **E** Developing fibrocollagenous
root sheath.
**A436.** Blonde, as there are no melanocytes in the precursor
epithelium.
see *Histology* p. 357

**A437. A Sebaceous gland**. The secretion of sebaceous glands
(sebum) is a lipid mixture, which includes triglycerides and
various complex waxes. It is produced by large scale necrosis of
the cells, resulting in release of their lipid content into the ducts
and thus into the space between the formed hair shaft and the
external root sheath, following degeneration of the internal root
sheath. This pattern of secretion is called 'holocrine' secretion;

**B Eccrine sweat gland and ducts**. Eccrine glands produce
sweat and are controlled by the autonomic nervous system.
Sweat is a hypotonic watery solution, with a neutral or slightly
acid pH, containing various ions, particularly sodium, potassium
and chloride ions;

**C Apocrine glands**. Apocrine glands produce a viscid, slightly
milky secretion in response to external stimuli such as fear,
sexual excitement, etc. The function of this secretion is not
known in man, but similar glands in mammals act as scent
organs for delineation of territory and sexual attraction.
see *Histology* p. 358-359

**A438.** Meissner's corpuscle.

**A439.** Detection of light touch.

**A440.** In the pulp of the fingers and toes, and around the nipples and lips.

see *Histology* p. 361

**A441.** Mammary lobule.

**A442.** Sexually mature female breast.

**A443.** **A** Intralobular terminal duct, **B** Terminal ductule (becomes secretory during pregnancy and lactation), **C** Intralobular fibrollagenous stroma, **D** Extralobular mammary adipose tissue.

**A444.** Fibroadenosis and cancer.

see *Histology* p. 367-368